BODYChange™

ALSO BY MONTEL WILLIAMS

A Dozen Ways to Sunday (with Daniel Paisner)

Life Lessons and Reflections

Mountain, Get Out of My Way!

Practical Parenting (co-authored with Jeffrey Gardère, Ph.D.)

℔ ℔ ℔

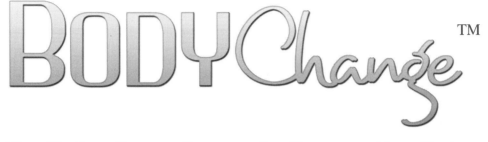

BODY Change™

The 21-Day Fitness Program for Changing Your Body
. . . and Changing Your Life!

MONTEL WILLIAMS

and

WINI LINGUVIC

MOUNTAIN
MOVERS
PRESS

an imprint of
Hay House, Inc.
Carlsbad, California • Sydney, Australia

Published and distributed in the United States by:
Mountain Movers Press, an imprint of Hay House, Inc., P.O. Box 5100, Carlsbad, CA 92018-5100 • (800) 654-5126 • (800) 650-5115 (fax) • www.hayhouse.com

Editorial supervision: Jill Kramer • *Design:* Summer McStravick
All interior photos (except for photo in Introduction): Mitchel Gray

Library of Congress Cataloging-in-Publication Data

Williams, Montel.
    BodyChange : the 21-day fitness program for changing your body — and changing your life! / Montel Williams and Wini Linguvic.
        p. cm.
    ISBN 1-58825-004-0
        1. Physical fitness—Handbooks, manuals, etc. 2. Exercise—Handbooks, manuals, etc. 3. Nutrition—Handbooks, manuals, etc. I. Title: Body Change. II. Linguvic, Wini. III. Title.

GV481 .W555 2001
613.7—dc21

                                                                    2001030038

ISBN 1-58825-004-0

04 03 02 01   6 5 4 3
1st printing, June 2001
3rd printing, August 2001

Printed in the United States of America

CONTENTS

• Acknowledgments •

I'd like to thank Wini for helping me look and feel better than ever. Angela Lee, Nancy Goldman, and Susan Schwartz for helping to harness our voices—this has truly been a group effort. Guy Rocourt for introducing me to snowboarding and helping me find great joy in what could have been my darkest hour. My family, friends, and staff, who are always there to support me. And most of all to my children, Ashley, Maressa, Montel II, and Wynter. My daily fight to stay healthy is based entirely on my desire to be able to enjoy our future together.

— Montel Williams

ℒ ℒ ℒ

My deepest thanks to the many wonderful people who have supported me, including Montel . . . thank you for sharing your story. Angela Lee and Melanie McLaughlin for believing in and guiding this project. My clients for their willingness to go beyond maintenance. My students, who teach me in every class. My family and friends for their love and encouragement. Special thanks to Kim Schwartz and Judy Greenbaum for teaching me about support.

My deepest gratitude to Janice Roven. Your love and friendship has always been my solid ground.

— Wini Linguvic

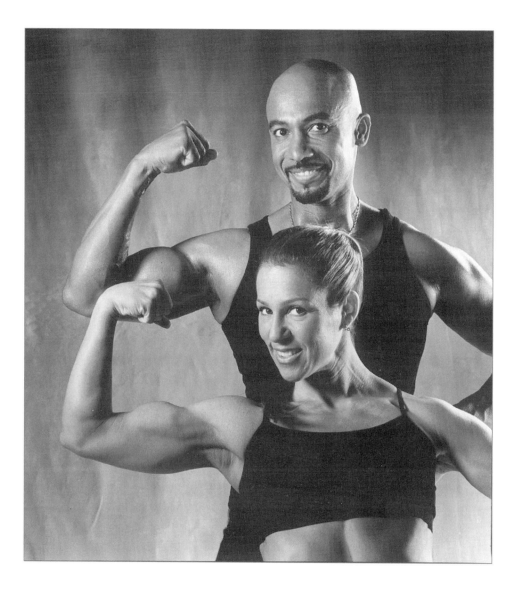

INTRODUCTION

by Montel Williams

The woman whose face you see, along with mine, right there on the cover of this book, and whose beautifully shaped body you'll see throughout these pages, is not some professional model that Mountain Movers Press found to entice you to purchase a workout book. This woman is not a gimmick or a phony. She's the real thing—my fitness trainer, Wini Linguvic, and the message she delivers about fitness in these pages will not only change your body, it will change your life. I guarantee it. Because it happened to me. Let me explain.

I've been training with Wini for the last four or five years, but I've known her a lot longer than that—she's a trainer at the gym I've gone to since I moved to New York nine years ago. The first thing I noticed about Wini, I've got to admit, were her legs. She has what are clearly the most beautiful; perfectly shaped; long, muscular legs that I've ever seen on any human being. But I noticed a lot more about Wini as I observed her in the gym most mornings. She had a focus and a determination about training that I didn't often see in anyone else at the gym. She was also quiet when she trained someone—soft-spoken and very intense.

If you've ever been fortunate enough to train in one gym at the same time of day over a period of years, you'll notice something that I see all the time: There are bodies there that come in regularly, do their workouts conscientiously, yet never change. Year after year, the people attached to those bodies come in, and they sweat and they lift weights, and I suppose they walk out feeling better, but you wouldn't know it from the way their bodies look. Maybe they go home after their workouts and eat a healthy breakfast and a good lunch and then wolf down a pint of Häagen-Dazs after dinner. I don't know. But I do know that whatever they're doing isn't improving their body shapes.

I noticed over the years that Wini's clients didn't look like most of those people I just described. I could definitely see improvements in the bodies of the people she trained, and I also saw that they were working with the same concentration and intensity I noticed in Wini. In the following pages, as Wini lays out her fitness philosophy and personal story, as well as her BodyChange fitness program, you'll come to understand why.

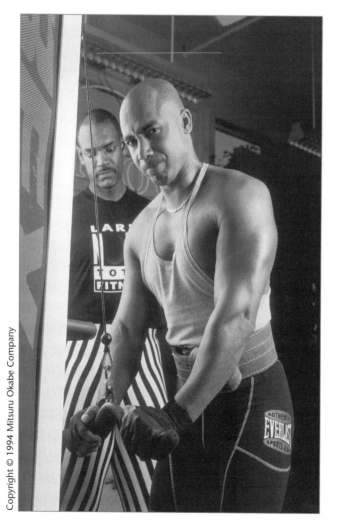

About five years ago, I found myself in a situation that, to my surprise, made me feel a bit uncomfortable. I was shooting a segment of the TV series *Matt Waters,* and in one scene I had to jump into a pool dressed in nothing but a pair of swim trunks. Now, despite my years of working out, I felt uneasy about appearing in front of a camera dressed in so little clothing. Don't get me wrong—at the time, I was very muscular and as physically fit as I wanted to be. And when I taped the talk show each week, dressed up in shirts and vests and sweaters and occasionally a suit, I felt fine about the shape I was in. But appearing in a dramatic TV series episode dressed in nothing but a swimsuit was a different matter. I wanted a leaner look—and I needed to get it quickly. So that's when I approached Wini.

Actually, I walked up to her and made some comment about her legs, like: "What on earth do you do for those thighs?" And from the way she reacted, I knew she understood I wasn't coming on to her. Not at all. I knew she could tell that I was speaking to her as one bodybuilder to another who wanted to know the secrets of the training plan that could produce legs like the ones she possessed. And from the way she answered, I knew I had found my trainer—someone who I'll keep training with for the next 10, 15, or 25 years, or as long as I'm able.

Wini told me about the BodyChange program, reinforcing my belief that changing your body is possible if you know how to do it correctly. Take a look at the photo of me from 1994 (on the previous page), when I posed for *Muscular Development* magazine, and compare it to any of the current photographs you see in this book. At that time, my training goals were quite different from the ones I have today. Then I was training for bulk, for size. I was perhaps 212 pounds in that photo, but muscular and fit, and I thought my six-foot frame handled that amount of weight well.

I told Wini about the TV episode and my upcoming role in it, and explained that I had three weeks to change my body shape to a leaner physique so that I would look better in a swimsuit. The time frame didn't faze her. All she needed to know was that I would be willing to work with her one hour a day, six days a week, with 100 percent concentration toward my stated goal of a leaner, buffer body. She promised she would help me get there. Wini's BodyChange fitness program is the same 21-day program that we're now sharing with you (modified for anyone's fitness level—even a beginner)!

Today I'm 192 pounds, and Wini and I refine my overall fitness goals every few months, and my more immediate goals every few days. We both just completed a training and diet regimen that produced the lean, cut bodies you see in this book's photos.

As I write this account of my fitness story, snowboarding season is upon us, and my training goals have changed again. Since my body will be bundled up on the slopes, the cut, highly chiseled look you see here is less important to me than the balance and coordination I'll need to control my snowboard. So we've added even more functional exercises, which you'll read about in subsequent chapters. By the time you read this book, my fitness goals will have changed again. Snowboarding season will be over, and tank-top season will be here. But I know with absolute certainty that, by using the BodyChange program, I'll achieve my new training goals.

By reading this book and following Wini's program, you may not become the next weightlifting champ or be able to run a marathon in under three hours, but you *will* see changes in your body, in your overall attitude, and in your life. The fitness program in this book will prepare you for what Wini calls "the sport of life," and you'll see the changes begin to occur in 21 days—as long as you firmly set your goals and dedicate yourself to making those objectives a reality. Whether your goal is to get up off that couch and walk up a flight of stairs more easily than you did yesterday, prepare for childbirth, recover from surgery, or see muscles you haven't seen in years, Wini's BodyChange program will not only train you, it will inspire you to make the changes you know you need to make.

After 21 days, the results you achieve will inspire you to set *new* goals and stick with them—and you'll experience for yourself the beauty of the BodyChange program. The benefits are yours for the asking.

ℓ ℓ ℓ

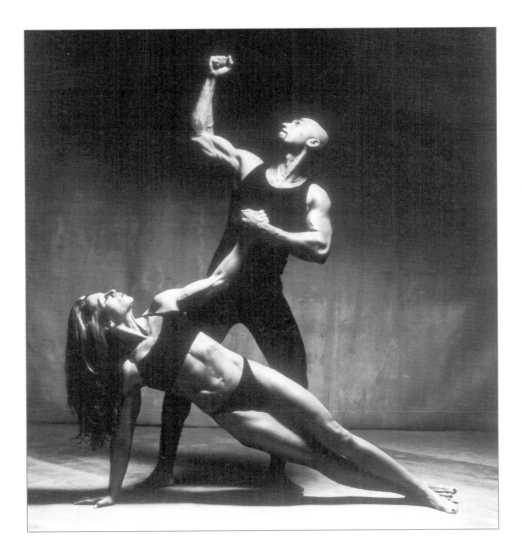

PART I

· The Program ·

CHAPTER 1

What Is the BodyChange Program?

When Montel first told me that he wanted me to write a workout book with him, I was ecstatic. I'd wanted to put my program on paper for years, and the fact that Montel is my dream client made the situation perfect. The big hurdle, then, was to put into words the actions that Montel and I go through daily, almost as routinely as we breathe. Here goes.

The BodyChange program is a 21-day exercise routine that incorporates aerobics, weight training, and core and functional exercises to improve your balance, coordination, and strength. In the sport of life, we need these attributes to face the challenges that are put in front of us, whether these challenges come to us at the gym, at work, or at home. If you follow the program for 21 days, you will not only feel better and see improvements in your body tone and your mood, but you'll get in the habit of moving, working out, and feeling good—and that habit will become a hard one to break. Then you'll want to set a new 21-day goal to keep the momentum going.

The BodyChange program relies less on big, complex machines and more on free weights, a bench, and what I call **core exercises.** The program can be done just as effectively at home as in a gym. The aerobics and weight-training exercises are straightforward, and are discussed in detail in Part II of this book. But what about attitude? That's the motivation that many of us—even hard-core trainers—have to develop and sustain in order to make changes in our routines and in our lives. Attitude is what enables us to move mountains, whether that mountain is a concrete goal ("I want to really impress my former classmates at my upcoming 20th high school reunion") or a vague plan ("I would love to be more active this summer").

Montel and I hope that, in reading about our efforts to move the mountains on the road to keeping fit, you too will see that whatever excuse you have for not training—or not training harder—will be exposed for exactly what it is: an excuse. We hope that you'll be able to better deal with whatever is keeping you *on* the couch and *off* your feet—even if it's a chronic, debilitating illness—and that somewhere in these pages, you'll find the keys that unlock a new attitude. If we succeed in merely getting you to *think* about your life in a different way, we'll consider our efforts in writing this book to be a success.

Beyond Maintenance

When was the last time you tested your limits? If you're like most people, it was probably when you took the physical fitness test in high school—or maybe that premed course in college. We tend to push ourselves early on, then kind of relax and forget how exhilarating improvement can be. Have you stretched yourself recently? I don't mean when you get up in the morning. What I mean is this: When was the last time you took on a truly challenging task at work, or sat down to have a difficult conversation with your partner, or spoke up in the face of adversity for a cause you believe in? Do you remember the last time you moved past your comfort zone into unfamiliar territory? We get so used to doing the easy thing that we forget that putting ourselves out there—whether beginning an exercise routine or falling in love—is what it truly means to be alive.

Challenges come into our lives in all kinds of packages. Right now, cross your arms. Did you put your right arm on top of your left? Try switching. Did you find the movement a little uncomfortable? It might take a little extra effort to remember to do it that way next time. At the very least, it would require some awareness.

The BodyChange program starts with awareness. You can't have change without awareness. What do you need to be aware of? First, that for the hour or so per day you engage in the exercise routine, you need to give it 100 percent of your attention. Second, you need to be aware that change can sometimes be uncomfortable. Third, you must believe that you have the power to change your body, and if you can change your body . . . you can change your life. As Montel says, you can even move mountains.

Training in Color

The core exercises of the BodyChange program may look simple, but don't be deceived. If you stay 100 percent aware while you perform them, you'll begin to notice amazing results in your body. We all have moments of being truly aware—watching our children sleep peacefully, or breathing in the fresh air, for example. So try to attain that level of awareness when you're lifting the weights—really *feel* what you're doing. Don't think about anything but the movement you're doing and what your body feels like.

It's not as easy as it sounds, yet it becomes easier with practice. It requires that you stay in the moment, or, as the Zen expression says, "feel your feet in your shoes." I call it **training in color.** Training in color is feeling the exercise fully—knowing that your muscles are fatigued after ten reps, yet doing the two more reps you're not so confident about. Those two reps are the really important ones. Soon, those two extra reps that require extra effort will become easier.

But back to being in the moment. How often are we *truly* present in the moment? Why don't you try this simple exercise right now: Put this book down (only for a moment!), then close your eyes and feel your feet—not by touching them, but by thinking about how they feel. Feel your knees, your legs . . . work your way up your body. Then consider this: What would it be like to feel your body while you're squeezing out those last two reps? If you're like me, probably a little uncomfortable. Awareness is demanding. While "feeling" your body in the above exercise, did you get distracted? Did your mind start to wander to the kids, the fridge, or the TV?

Here's an important question: At what point did you become distracted? Being aware of *when* you become distracted during an exercise is a good starting point for determining the kind of changes you need to make. I've noticed that being aware can be a real metaphor for life. Do you get distracted when something becomes difficult? If so, does that motivate you to try harder or to give up? Do you become distracted when something is too easy? If that's the case, do you get bored and disconnect, or do you look for ways to increase the challenge set before you? How do you avoid feelings of discomfort? Some people reach for a bag of cookies or a six-pack of beer. Others go shopping or gamble. How do *you* make life easier? Did you ever consider that staying with the discomfort—truly feeling it and not avoiding it—will, in the long run, make you stronger?

Incorporating Change

Change—any kind of change—is uncomfortable, particularly as we get older. Many people I know are stuck in jobs they dislike because they're afraid of change. They would rather suffer their familiar discomfort than chart unknown waters. BodyChange teaches you how to be "comfortably uncomfortable." The program starts by saying, "You're stronger than you think." But to experience that strength, you've got to stretch beyond that feeling of comfort—what I call "training outside your comfort zone"—to test where your limits are and expand what feels comfortable to you. Once you *do* expand your comfort zone, you'll then begin to notice small but significant changes in your body, in your attitude, and in your life.

Part of the message of this book is *don't underestimate yourself.* One of Montel's mottos is: "There is nothing on this planet I cannot do." I once asked him if he was scared or uncomfortable the first time he spoke before an audience. His answer was amazing: "Absolutely. I *still* get anxious." So each time he has to appear, he sets his mind to it and works through the discomfort. If he hadn't confronted his fear of speaking before an audience, if he hadn't worked through his discomfort, he would never be where he is today.

In the gym, I teach my clients to seek out that point of discomfort, to embrace it as their next challenge. Where there's that sticking point, there's also an opportunity to get stronger.

If you're still uncomfortable about being uncomfortable, think about this: It really hurts more to stay in the same place, to *not* challenge yourself. If you don't believe me, then *stop* trying to improve. Stop trying to reach your potential. Tell me *that* doesn't hurt! Not meeting your potential has to be the most uncomfortable feeling of all.

Montel certainly understands this concept. In fact, he's written an entire book called *Mountain, Get Out of My Way,* about his efforts to deal with the challenges that he has confronted on his path, and later in these pages, he'll explain how that concept is not only related to being physically fit, but is utterly relevant to his entire life today.

Believe in Yourself

Once you realize that you can change your body, you can move mountains. We've already established that you need to work at a 100 percent effort level, but most people dislike that kind of discomfort and intensity. BodyChange says that once you commit to working hard and accept being temporarily "comfortably uncomfortable," in 21 days you'll see definite changes in your body. And it goes a step further, because once you see changes in your body, you'll start to believe in yourself and find inner strength in other areas of your life as well.

Those feelings of strength and control will motivate you to continue using and adapting the BodyChange program. Montel comes to the gym every day because of the little accomplishments he achieves each time he's there. It's those little successes that motivate him to try harder on each successive day.

Don't get me wrong, failures can be motivating, too, but which feels better? While working out, you only have yourself to rely on. Even if you have the best trainer in the world, you still have to do the work yourself. There's no neighbor, friend, or therapist to help you through the drill—no ex-lover or boss to blame if you don't complete it. It's just you and the weights. But on the flip side, the accomplishments you achieve are all yours. You've earned them, and no one can take them away from you. You carry them with you throughout the day and throughout your life.

Montel and I find that control over our fate—even for that one hour in the gym most mornings—is very reassuring. We know that we're responsible for our own bodies—how they look and feel. Others may find this kind of control very daunting. It would be much easier to place the responsibility for our successes or failures (in the gym) on our parents (for their genes), on our partner (for keeping those cookies in the house), on our colleagues (for ordering pizza for lunch), or on our friends (for persuading us to go out for a few beers). But by giving away that responsibility, we're also giving away our power. Montel and I accept the responsibility and use our power to create and recreate ourselves. Trust me, there are days we slip, days that we go to the gym but we're just not up to the task. But we don't beat ourselves up about it. Instead, we remember our successes and how good it felt to follow the BodyChange program—and that's what gets us back on track.

The journey to fitness is a process, and it's an exciting experience to push yourself and find out what you're capable of. My clients love the results they get from their workouts. They come to the gym ready to work, and keep up with their programs because they enjoy pushing beyond their previous limits. There's no denying that the BodyChange program is a challenge, making not only physical demands but mental and emotional ones, too. But think of it this way: Won't it feel good to do something that truly challenges you, and effects change not only in your body, but in your mind and soul as well?

As you prepare to embark on the BodyChange program, you might find it helpful to understand why Montel and I decided to write this book. By seeing where we've come from in some detail and how we use the BodyChange program to achieve results, you'll see how this program can help *you* make significant changes in your own life.

ℰ ℰ ℰ

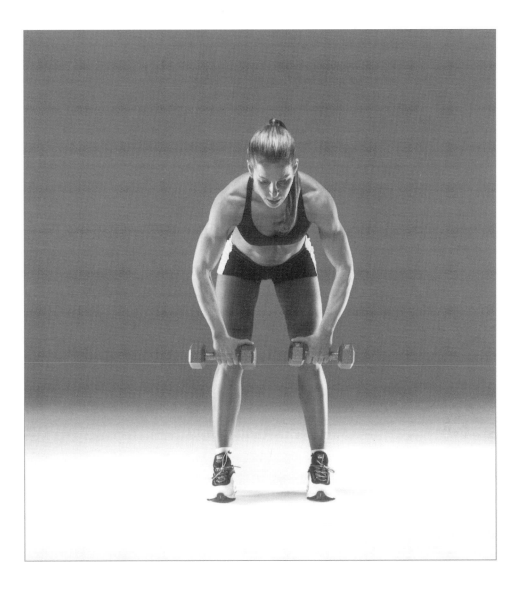

CHAPTER 2

A Word from Montel: Mountain, Get Out of My Way!

I've exercised almost every day since I was 16. It's like brushing my teeth. There have been brief periods when I've stopped—those times when my schedule has gotten so ridiculous that I simply didn't have a moment to get to a gym, or times when for a week or so I was down with a cold or the flu. For example, when I spent months and months on-board submarines during my service in the Navy, there was literally no place to exercise, even though I wanted to. But I always got back to my fitness routine. And I have to tell you that I've always felt better after each workout. Absolutely. But how can I convince *you* of that?

I've been athletic since I was a kid. In high school, I started performing in a band and wanted to stay in shape to look good on stage. When I joined the service, the military emphasized fitness, but by that time, I was training a step beyond what was required. For instance, if they required 10 push-ups, I would do 20. My attitude was, why stop at 20 if I could do 25? That's just the way I am. I don't want to be on the playing field if I can't play my hardest. I've always felt that if I'm not giving 100 percent, then I'm just wasting my time. I'm that way with exercise, with my talk show, with raising my kids, and dealing with my chronic illness, multiple sclerosis (MS).

I know that many of you view exercise as something you'll do tomorrow, or something that seems too difficult to attempt. Some of you may exercise regularly, yet you don't notice much change in your body from month to month or year to year, and you aren't exactly sure what to do about it.

Well, this is the way I think about fitness: All I have in this life is me. If I can't motivate *me,* who can? When I'm not the best I can be, I feel lousy because I know deep inside that I could have done better. But when I leave the gym having accomplished one little thing—something as simple as one extra rep that I hadn't been able to do the day before—then I know that I've pushed myself and made myself better today than I was yesterday. I've expanded my limitations, stepped out of what Wini calls my "comfort zone," and gone beyond maintenance into the place where change happens. If I do one more rep today, I can do two more next week or next month.

Will those changes take work? Definitely. Will they take time? Probably. But the fact is that by doing just one more rep, or adding an extra two-and-a-half pounds to my workout, I've just learned that I can change. And if I can change how much weight I lift, or how many times I can lift it, I can change my body. I know it's a leap of faith, but if I can change my body, I can change the way I negotiate a business deal, spend time with my kids, and cope with a debilitating disease—all those things in life that really matter.

You see, it's not just about changing your body—that's just where it starts. It's about changing your attitude. If Wini and I accomplish nothing more in this book, I hope we change your *attitude* about fitness.

Six days a week, I go to the gym to feel empowered. I like to begin my day, every day, with the feeling that I've accomplished something, even before I get into my office or hit the studio. The thing that made me want to train with Wini was her BodyChange program's philosophy: "What do I have to do at the gym to help me perform better in the sport of life?" Wini knew that the gym wasn't an end, but a means—a means to feeling better about myself so that I could be more effective in *all* aspects of my life.

• • •

I entered the service at the age of 17, and as almost everybody knows, physical fitness is a key element of military life. Staying physically fit in the military is not a choice, it's a requirement. In the Marine Corps boot camp, I scored the maximum on the physical fitness test every time I was required to take it. I entered the Naval Academy at age 20 and took up boxing. At this point in my life, I was a 147-pound welterweight. I turned to weight lifting after I was forced to quit boxing due to a knee injury. Within a year, I had gained more than 30 pounds of muscle. Needless to say, my six-foot frame was much better suited to my new 180-pound physique.

After graduating from the Naval Academy, I was stationed in Guam and really got the bodybuilding bug. I started power lifting at a ferocious rate. I packed on another 30-plus pounds of muscle and began competing. I took third place in the 1981 Mr. Guam contest and second place in the 1981 Mr. Far East Military competition. After Guam, I began spending a lot of time at sea. On-board a surface ship, there's usually some sort of makeshift gym, but on-board a submarine, there's simply no place to work out. So I tried to get creative by lifting garbage cans and gear lockers.

In my early 30s, I was constantly traveling. I went all over the country speaking to more than three million teenagers about staying off drugs and staying in school. During this period of my life, if I couldn't find a nearby gym, I would ask the high schools to let me use their gymnasiums after the students had gone home. So I was able to keep in shape, even during the grueling travel schedule I had to keep up.

In 1991, those lectures to the kids led to the development of my talk show, which is heading into its 11th season on the air. In the early days, I was spending 16 hours a day producing and taping the show. We've been successful, added staff, and refined the process a bit so that the 16-hour days are confined to a mere three or four a week. A normal person might take the well-deserved time and relax a bit, but I'm now acting in, directing, and producing TV programs and films. However, I still find time to train with Wini most mornings. As you might guess, I don't accept anyone's excuse that they don't have time to exercise. There's always time if you make your workout enough of a priority to schedule it in.

In 1999, at age 43, I was diagnosed with MS, and since then I've been adapting to its unpredictable, insidious symptoms. The doctors gave me their conventional wisdom: *Take it easy. Find ways to eliminate stress from your life.* But those doctors didn't know who they were dealing with. Denying me my strenuous workouts would be like denying me air to breathe. The MS diagnosis was just one more mountain I had to push out of my way. For me, the only way to do so was to work out. And I find that, after doing one of Wini's workouts first thing in the morning, there is no stress that the rest of my day could present to me that I can't handle. I'm prepared for whatever mountain appears in my path, and I'm eager to knock it out of my way.

The sport of my life has been different for each of those periods, and so has my body. The workout I do today is different from the one I did yesterday or five months ago or five years ago, because the way I spend my life is different today. And it will be different tomorrow. What won't be different is my attitude, my intensity, and the confidence that I can do anything I set my mind to.

The point I'm trying to make is this: You don't have to have my same training goals to achieve dramatic changes in your body and in your fitness level. In fact, I assume most of you *don't* have these same goals. But I'm willing to bet anything that you *do* want to make changes in your body. To do that, you'll have to set goals that are appropriate for you, and be willing to work toward them—no matter what they are and what it takes to achieve them.

Look at me. I'm almost 45, and I think I look better today than I did a decade ago. I have a chronic illness that keeps trying to stop me from doing the things I love, but despite it, I directed my first film, wrote three books, recently celebrated my tenth season on the air, and even took up snowboarding. I couldn't have done all of that if Wini's BodyChange program hadn't shown me that small daily accomplishments lead to big changes—in your body and in your life.

You've heard me talk about the obstacles that get between us and our goals in life, and you probably know that I believe most of the obstacles are ones we create for ourselves. What are the obstacles *you've* put in the way of getting physically fit?

Defining the Mountain

When it comes to getting in shape, I've heard all the excuses:

"I'll start working out tomorrow."
"Sticking to a fitness routine is too hard."
"I just don't have time to exercise."
"I get enough of a workout running after the kids all day."
"I have an old injury that prevents me from keeping fit."
"I'm so out of shape that I might have a heart attack if I start exercising now."
"Exercising is just so boring!"
"I just had a baby and I'm exhausted."
"I'm recovering from surgery and can't do much in terms of getting fit."
"I have a chronic illness that prevents me from taxing my system."

The list goes on and on, and it's a list I'm familiar with, because the excuses on this list have been voiced, at some point or other, by almost everyone—even by me. Sure, there are days when I get out of bed that I don't feel like getting myself to the gym. But as Wini always tells me, those are precisely the days that it's most important for me to get myself there.

Because of the way I'm affected by MS, there are days when I essentially have to rewire my brain before I can rise from bed, then put one foot in front of the other to get myself to the bathroom and brush my teeth. This process can take me 15 or 20 minutes. Having MS would be an excellent excuse for not working out, wouldn't it? But I know that this mountain of chronic illness was put in my path for a reason, and I'm determined to shove that excuse right out of my way. Why? Because I know that my workouts provide the balance I need to offset the challenges MS presents me with each day. I keep that in mind on those dark winter mornings when I don't want to get up and do my workout.

How do you define the mountain that is keeping *you* from getting physically fit? Which of the excuses listed above most accurately describes the mountain you're facing on the road to feeling and looking better?

Setting Goals

Here's the secret to moving that mountain: You must set a goal that lies on the other side of it. Your fitness goals are your own. I can't presume to tell you where you need to be in terms of your own performance and conditioning. Only *you* have answers to those questions. But I can guarantee you that, until you search for and then set definite goals—with a definite timetable for achieving them—that mountain will stay right there in the middle of your pathway.

That's where BodyChange comes in. You start by setting a very specific goal: "I want thinner thighs!" "I want to lose a dress size!" "I want to lose an inch from my waist!" Make sure it's something you can accomplish in 21 days. You might *want* to lose three dress sizes, but for now, just focus on dropping that first one.

After the word got out that I was writing this book, I got a call from *Muscle and Fitness* magazine asking me to do a photo shoot. Now, it was the middle of winter, and I was spending every nonworking minute on my snowboard. I was thrilled to do the shoot, but I asked for three weeks. This time my specific 21-day BodyChange goal was to put on three to five pounds of rock-hard muscle. I buckled down and focused.

How do you accomplish a goal like this? You must first take stock of your fitness history. Perhaps you've never worked out a day in your life, or you haven't since playing field hockey in high school or volleyball on the beach last summer. Or, at the other end of the spectrum, perhaps you've been going to a gym for a few months or even a few years, but aren't happy with the results you're getting. I see it all the time: people who work out regularly, but whose bodies never seem to change. And what I notice is that these are the people who are focused on everything *but* their workout routines while they're at the gym. They'll read while sitting on an adductor machine, or zone out on the treadmill watching the TV monitor for the latest stock market quotes. Some are more interested in catching up with the latest neighborhood gossip than doing what they came to the gym to do: work out!

Using the BodyChange program, it doesn't matter what your fitness level is when you begin. The point of setting your fitness goal is to know where you want to be 21 days after you start. Your goal should be realistic and achievable. You don't want to set yourself up for failure. If you haven't exercised since high school, let's be real—in 21 days you won't be ready to run a marathon. Perhaps your 21-day goal will be to get off the couch and walk up a flight of stairs without becoming as winded as you did today.

Has simple inertia been your mountain, your obstacle to getting fit for the last 15 or 20 years of your life? Or has it been your demanding job or problems with your kids? You know what I think? I think you need to get off the sofa and start a workout routine. In these matters, I subscribe to the school of small victories. By that I mean that I earn a small victory every day from my sense of having accomplished something. If you can get through the first workout by yourself—even if it's three days later that you get through that workout again—you've had two accomplishments in a week that you wouldn't have had before.

How do I motivate you to set 21-day goals and start achieving them? I can't, really. If motivation came in a bottle, everyone would have some. But I can share what I've learned from personal experience: It's a matter of consistency. That's the reason I recommend Wini's BodyChange program. It's only 21 days long. *Try it for 21 days.* What do you have to lose? By the time you get to the 21st day, I guarantee you that your attitude toward working out will change to the point where you feel that it's a part of your life, because, quite simply, the changes you see and the way you feel *will* become a habit. Not only that, but I suspect you'll miss it if you slack off for a couple of days or don't do it altogether.

After the first 21 days, you'll be encouraged to set a new fitness goal for the *next* 21 days. Pretty soon, working out six days a week will be as natural to you as getting out of bed in the morning. If you can make your workout a habit, or if you can learn to intensify the workout you've been doing for years, you'll have moved a mountain right out of your way.

Passive vs. Active Living

Let me tell you something you'll appreciate: When you opened up the pages of this book, you moved your first mountain. You indicated a willingness to overcome the inertia that has kept you from achieving your fitness goals. After you set your first 21-day fitness goal, you will have moved your second mountain. This process reminds me of my version of the old saying, "Being in the right place at the right time." I say, "Make every place the right place all the time." Someone who lives passively waits for things to happen. Someone actively engaged in life makes those things happen that will enhance their life.

How does this apply to fitness? The BodyChange program requires a focused intensity on each step of the routine. Not only does Wini ask you to feel the muscle you're exercising, she challenges you to feel it **in color!** What she means is that she wants you to put all your mental and physical energy into the one rep, that one set of exercises that you're doing at the moment. She challenges you to exercise actively to get the best results. Sitting on a machine, reading while doing reps—even if that were possible—won't get you anywhere, just as passive living won't get you any closer to your life's goals.

It's a matter of taking action. I'm a person who believes that the only way to live is to push that coin off the edge of the desk—I'm not going to sit still. So every single day of my life, I'm pushing toward something that I hope will create something better.

You may not think you possess whatever it takes to push that envelope, to live actively rather than passively, so here's where the BodyChange program can help: You set your 21-day goal, however modest it is, and make sure you achieve it. Then you set another 21-day goal, and make sure you achieve that one, too. Pretty soon, goal setting in your life becomes as natural as breathing. It becomes a habit that's hard to break. Training in your home or in the gym is training for the sport of life. The good news is that the skills and discipline you pick up from working out transfer to all areas: family, work, spirituality, interpersonal interactions, and more!

Proactive Exercise

It follows, then, that the BodyChange program requires you to be proactive about your exercise routine. That means recognizing that every single exercise, every single rep, and every single set counts toward achieving your goal! Even if you increase your intensity by as little as two-and-a-half pounds over a period of time, remember: That's two-and-a-half pounds you couldn't lift before. You don't want to take it easier on the last set. If it's going to be a challenge anyway, why not try it? As Wini will explain, we need to go outside our comfort zones—we need to move that mountain that's in our way so real change can begin.

Sure, you're going to get sore. The only thing to do then is *move!* If you're too sore to do a squat, take a walk. The only way to get the lactic acid out of your muscles is to get the blood pumping through them.

A Note on Chronic Disease

Perhaps the most formidable mountain that any of us can face on our road to keeping fit is that of living with a chronic disease, whether it's the MS that's wreaking havoc on my body and those of millions of people around the world, the asthma that some of us develop in childhood or beyond, different types of diabetes, hepatitis C, or a real bizarre one—sarcoidosis—which my friend Revlon model Karen Duffy is coping with. How we deal with these types of challenges very much reflects the way we deal with many other aspects of our lives. Forgive me for getting personal, but I've learned a lot in the two years since my diagnosis, and perhaps my experience can help those of you living with chronic disease—and your loved ones—cope just a little bit better.

As those of you who have illness as a constant companion know, receiving the diagnosis is a life-changing event. It can leave you shattered, angry, depressed, or even worse—full of despair. You don't mean to, but sometimes you can't help but take your feelings out on the people closest to you, the very ones you're going to need to help you cope. Those first few days or weeks can be truly wrenching. But then you begin to realize, *Hey! I'm still me. I've got the wherewithal to deal with everything. Let's start!* And you usually try to find out everything there is to know about living with your disease.

As I mentioned above, although things are changing rapidly, the conventional wisdom that doctors impart to people diagnosed with MS is to rest, reduce stress, and be careful not to raise the body's temperature for too long a time. Physical activity is certainly recommended for anyone who can perform it, for as long as they are able (the course the disease takes on the body is unpredictable), but in moderation.

No high-intensity aerobic workouts that go on forever and raise the body temperature for long periods of time. That's the conventional wisdom.

I knew that advice wouldn't work for me, though. After the initial shock wore off, I was determined to live as actively and as intensely as I always had for as long as I could. I discussed this with my doctors, and Wini and I approached the gym as a way to enhance my day, to improve the quality of my life. We really cranked up my workouts. My illness is definitely one of my extra motivating factors, and the reason why I work out as intently and intensely as I do.

Intensity is a relative term. It's personal to the individual, just as goals are. My goal happens to be that I'm going to be as fit as I can possibly be. MS is *not* going to stop me in any way, shape, or form. Other people will have different training goals, so their level of intensity will be aligned with their own objectives in the gym. They will work intensely the entire time, but their intensity may not be the same as mine. I am intense in every aspect of my life. I can be intense to a fault, I guess, in some ways, but I'm intense about *everything*. But you know what? It's really just like passion. You can live your life passionless, or you can live your life *full of* passion. I choose the latter.

Since one side of my body is more affected by the disease than the other, Wini and I have been concentrating on functional exercises—the lunges, push-ups, squats, and so forth—that require balance, coordination, and strength—the same exercises that are described later in this book. I believe our approach has been so successful that most people can't tell from my appearances on the talk show, or when they meet me in person, how I'm being challenged by the disease.

To put my situation into perspective, and to use the metaphor I've been asking you to think about, MS is just one more mountain I've had to move to live the life I'm determined to live. As many of you who have read my memoir know, I was born into a family that worked hard and did well, but we faced racism throughout our lives. It's out there, it's a mountain I had to learn how to move, and I've been quite successful in my life because I never let that mountain be an obstacle to my achievements.

I had to work my way through school and face the prospect of being the first black enlisted Marine to graduate from the Naval Academy Prep School, and then go on to graduate from the Naval Academy in Annapolis. And my challenges didn't stop there—they started there. No, I didn't have to be a Marine or go to the Naval Academy; I would have excelled at a community college. I didn't have to push myself to the point that I was awarded the Armed Forces Expeditionary Medal, two Navy Expeditionary Medals, two Humanitarian Service Medals, a Navy Achievement Medal, two Navy Commendation Medals, and two Meritorious Service Awards. I guess I could have just "cruised" through. But that's not who I am. The one time I felt I didn't give life my best shot was at the Naval Academy. I worked hard, but always had the gnawing suspicion that I could have worked harder and even done better.

Now how does this life experience apply to fitness and chronic disease? Well, I learned an important lesson from my time at the Academy. Instead of moving mountains there, I was satisfied to "coast" along, just below the summit. But that process didn't feel good, and I've kept that in mind every day since I graduated. I decided that the only way I wanted to get through life was as an active player. I promised myself I would always raise the bar, elevate my standards, and expect nothing short of excellence from myself and from those around me. I tried to convey that attitude when I spoke to high school students in the early 1990s. If I changed one young life—persuaded one kid to stay off drugs and stay in school—among all those who attended my presentations, then I consider my efforts to have been a success.

It's the same standard that I apply to my fitness routine. I expect excellence from myself, and I always try to achieve it. Despite the challenges to my body as a result of having MS, I refuse to let the disease stand in my way. Excellence is the standard by which I live life and by which I train.

If you're coping with a chronic disease, listen to your doctor, but also listen to your heart. Push as hard as you can by setting the kinds of 21-day goals you'll learn about in the BodyChange program. Once physical activity—performed to the highest standard of which you are capable—becomes a habit, there's no feeling like it in the world. The rush you get from performing the best workout you know how to do will carry you through some pretty dark days. Trust me. I know because I've been there, and all I wish for you is the strength to do your best.

ﻤ ﻤ ﻤ

CHAPTER 3

Wini's Story

A page from Wini's diary:

> 5:30 A.M.—my favorite time to train. I'll take care of the things I need to take care of later. This is <u>my</u> time. My workout. I work it in sometimes at strange hours depending on my schedule. The days when I don't have the time are the days I make sure to find the time.
>
> I don't need crowds of people around. I just need a gym and my music. My training is for me. I turn down the volume in the world and dial in to how I feel. Finally something not complicated: work hard=feel good.
>
> I search for the effort. I look for the point where I can't complete the rep. At least I can't complete it <u>today</u>. Today's work prepares me for tomorrow.
>
> I compare myself to who I was yesterday. Am I better? Am I stronger?
>
> I have another day of pushing myself beyond maintenance. Another training session to pile on top of the other training sessions. I recall all the workouts—and they stack one on top of the other—reminding me of how strong I've become. As I recall all the workouts I've done, I remember the times I went to the gym even if I was overwhelmed with trivia. The days I hit the gym to celebrate, and the times I hit the weights because I had to hit SOMETHING. I stand tall with the knowledge I can go beyond maintenance. <u>IT'S NOT JUST MY BODY I'VE BUILT IN THE GYM.</u>

I've been training for as long as I can remember. I don't remember not having a quest to better myself—as a person, an athlete, a student, or a teacher. I've used the gym to get me through my ups and downs.

It's the sense of control that's the best thing about working out. You feel as if you have some say in how you feel and how you look. You learn that you're strong, that you can dig in and work and see the benefits of that work. You know there are mountains, yet after a workout, the mountains that are in your way seem climbable. And if they're not, well, just blast a hole right through them!

I discovered the joys of working out when I was 16 years old. That's when I bought my first weight set. I had picked up a book by a woman named Lisa Lyon. This was before there were many weight-training books for women. I wanted to learn more, so I read Arnold Schwarzenegger's book *Arnold: The Education of a Bodybuilder.* I then proceeded to buy every fitness book out there.

But just reading about it wasn't enough. I wasn't interested in bodybuilding and fitness as a *spectator* sport. I wanted to find something physical that I could do. I wasn't athletic as a child. I spent much more time reading than playing on teams, so I wanted to somehow become an athlete as a young adult. I wanted to find an activity that I could participate in that had nothing to do with being on a team or playing against someone else. In that way, I could progress as quickly or as slowly as I wanted to. I wanted to compete against *myself,* with the victory being progress. There could be no second place if I did my best.

And like every other 16-year-old, I wanted to look better. So often we look to someone else to define what's beautiful. Working out helped me create my own definition of *beautiful.* Working out was something that made me believe in myself. Qualities such as independence, strength, and confidence appealed to my sense of beauty (although the search for the perfect lipstick continues).

I never set myself up to be like the Olympic athletes I would see on TV, or the professional bodybuilders I saw in the magazines; however, I took their efforts as a form of inspiration and decided to see what I could do myself. I competed in bodybuilding, had a blast, and took the discipline and lessons everywhere I went. I learned that training works. In the gym, I got back what I put in. In the gym, I realized, life was fair.

Developing the BodyChange Program

I've been working with clients for more than 15 years, and I know that this program works. People from various walks of life, with a variety of fitness goals, have changed their lives by incorporating exercise into their daily routine. The discipline that we slowly accumulate as the workouts pile up is priceless, and we bring our attitude from the gym out into the world. The confidence earned through hard work in the gym doesn't go away when your workout is over.

The BodyChange program developed over time as I saw results in my clients. Over the years, I kept the techniques and equipment that worked and discarded the rest—even if it was trendy. I discovered that there was no need to use every machine in the gym. Doing lunges across the floor generated better results than the fancy new leg machines. As I worked with my clients over time, the results of their hard work and commitment became evident. I found that people kept coming back for more training—not only because they looked great, but also because they enjoyed the workouts. The training hour was their time, and buff biceps or not, it was enjoyable.

I've been in the fitness business since I was 18 years old, and the results of people changing their lives—not just their bodies—is what keeps me going. Throughout the years, I've expanded the BodyChange program, incorporating the best elements of many fitness philosophies, combining them with the life lessons I've learned from being in the gym, and developing the program you'll find in these pages.

Today I work with my clients to develop a program that works for them. I take into account each person's present fitness level, the number of times a week that an individual can train, and that person's own long- and short-term fitness goals. If we decide to work together, I then design a program tailor-made for that man or woman. The reason why people stick with the BodyChange program is because it's the smartest exercise program they've found, and it offers them the right attitude about fitness. Even those who disliked working out in the past start to enjoy their time in the gym.

As I worked with people, I learned that it was not only the right training program that I gave them, but I was also able to share my passion for pushing them past their comfort zones into the area where real changes came quickly. That attitude kept people coming back to the workouts because they liked the way they felt, and they found that they liked themselves more—they were creating a new and different way to live.

When you teach someone to enjoy something—something that feels good and brings about results—adherence comes naturally.

℩ ℩ ℩

CHAPTER 4

The BodyChange Philosophy

The BodyChange program, as outlined in this book, describes basic exercises grouped into three categories (**core, functional,** and **weight training**). You will also be choosing certain aerobic activities to perform in conjunction with these exercises. The BodyChange program can be tailored to your own fitness level and goals. I'm assuming that each reader of this book begins at a different fitness level and has different training goals. Therefore, I recommend that everyone start at the beginner level. If you're familiar with weight-training routines and body-building techniques, you can advance rapidly to the next level, but you need to be proficient in all areas of the program. Believe it or not, I've trained marathon runners who could not do five push-ups. Some people simply have physical limitations and can't do certain exercises. That's why this program gives you options to tailor your routine to match your abilities and goals.

There are some core principles for all fitness programs. These beliefs include the importance of functional exercises, of strengthening the abdominals and lower back muscles (the core exercises), and of weight training for both women and men. These concepts are woven into a program that meets an individual's needs. Throughout these pages, you'll be able to design your own program. Weight training, strengthening the body's core, and functional exercises are essential to fitness, and they're the basis of the BodyChange program.

• • •

Montel: Wini's BodyChange program stops making exercise scary and breaks it down to its basic elements: free weights, functional exercises, abs, and back—and let's not forget intensity. In this section of the book, we explain how to reorient your entire approach to working out by starting you with the basic tools you'll need to do your first exercises. What else do you need? You need emotional intensity. You need to be focused. You need to resist placing limitations on your body before you even know what your limitations are. As Wini explains, you need to go beyond maintenance, beyond what feels familiar to you . . . into some uncharted territory. That's the difference between the BodyChange program and others you've tried or read about. It's not about one or two exercises; it's not about one or two gimmicks; it's not about one or two gadgets. And it's not just about 21 days. It's about the first 21 days, seeing the changes take place right before your eyes, and then setting a goal for another 21 days—moving one little mountain at a time.

The Basic Exercises That Achieve Results

In the gym, we need to work our muscles the way they were meant to be used as we go about our daily tasks—standing, lunging, bending, and squatting. The sport of life happens in motion. That's why you'll find that the exercises I recommend simulate real-life movements. These movements are designed to challenge your muscles to work together while promoting good posture. By using exercises that require motion through space, we present our body with an additional puzzle to which it must find a solution. If we learn how to balance as we lift our own body's weight up on one leg, or travel through space holding additional weights, our bodies will automatically use our abdominals, learn coordination, and correct our posture. I call these movements that require you to balance and guide your body weight through a range of motion **functional exercises.** They are basic to the BodyChange program.

Fitness training is not only about sculpted muscles, although they're a nice benefit. It's more about how much power your muscles can generate to move you through the sport of life, when you're not working out per se, either at home or in the gym. Functional training is a tool to make you a better athlete—whether you're swinging a golf club, conquering a hill on a bike, or carrying your toddler up a flight of stairs. Another advantage of functional exercises is that you don't need any special equipment to perform them. You don't even need to go to a gym. All you need is a description of how to perform the exercises correctly, and then an understanding of which muscles are being trained and what benefit you'll get out of doing the movements properly. I explain more about the functional exercises in Part II, where I describe the BodyChange exercises in detail.

When executing functional exercises, we choose movements in our workout routine that simulate movements that we do in our daily lives. My advanced clients like to do side lunges, for example, which are a good simulation of a common movement we perform on the tennis court when reaching for a passing shot. Passing a medicine ball to a partner, if done properly, can train your muscles, joints, and tendons for an aggressive game of beach volleyball or for lifting bags of groceries into the back of an SUV.

Walking lunges, which look easy but are extremely challenging to perform correctly, not only strengthen our thigh muscles, but help us achieve the kind of balance we need to grab a small child who's about to chase a ball into a busy street. Sport, whether on the tennis court or on a street corner, requires strength, balance, and a transfer of power from one side of our body to another—from the bottom of our feet to the top of our heads. Functional exercises provide strength in motion. And what good is strength if it can't be used in our day-to-day lives?

Also basic to the BodyChange program are those exercises that strengthen the core muscles: the abs and lower back. These muscles stabilize the power centers of our bodies. I'm a nut about strong abdominals, in particular, so you'll find many variations of crunches in these pages. Because so many of us have become sedentary, working long hours in front of a computer screen or relaxing in front of the TV screen at night, we forget these basic body skills.

A savvy freelance book editor I know kept telling me what a fabulous year she was having with her business, but what neither of us realized—until she began to have shooting pains down her legs and in her lower back—was that as part of her heavy workload, she was spending long hours sitting in front of her computer. She had always worked out, and she had always been fit, so it never occurred to me that she was cutting back on her exercise routine. The odd thing was that until she woke up one morning with excruciating pain in her lower back, she hadn't realized it either. In her drive to accomplish all that she had to do, she had forgotten to do her sit-ups every day.

After three weeks of almost total immobility, she realized the error of her ways and began to exercise her abs and lower back—gently at first, but then with an intensity she'd never had before. Now, she tells me, she's at her local gym at least six days a week, and half of the time that she's there is spent stretching out her lower back muscles and doing sit-up variations. (And whenever I e-mail her, I remind her to get to the gym no matter what her deadlines look like.) She reports that her once-aching back has never felt stronger.

The abdominals are special, which is why I elaborate on them so much. They're more difficult to feel than other muscles, and therefore more difficult to train. You can *see* a bicep working, but you have to put your hand on your stomach to feel your abs working. Think about the last time you did a set of sit-ups. Some people I know do crunches forever, and the only fatigue they ever feel is in their necks. If you do crunches correctly, you shouldn't be able to do many of them, and every single rep has to count.

I'm often asked what the difference is between core exercises and functional exercises. The distinction is important. Core exercises are those that work your abdominals and lower back, what I (and what most people) consider your *core*. In dancing, it's sometimes called your center. So, core exercises are those that focus on your abs and lower back. In addition to working your abs and lower back muscles, functional exercises also work your legs and move you through space. In these exercises, your abs and lower back muscles are stabilizing your body, but they're not the prime mover, the way they are when you're doing a crunch. In a functional exercise, the abdominals stabilize the center of the body as you move through space, but many other muscle groups are moving you from one place to another. Functional exercises integrate many muscle groups and involve more complex movements than core exercises.

The Mind-set: Beyond the Physical

Knowing which exercises to do and how to perform them well is important, but just as important is your attitude toward your workout. The BodyChange program is not just about looking buff. Looking good is important, but we demand more by asking, *What can I do?* rather than *How do I look?* Can I give myself a challenge by saying, *I need to do this,* and then by doing it? Can I take myself beyond where I am today to a place I've never been before? If necessary, can I be a beginner again and take up an entirely new fitness challenge?

I recently set a new challenge for myself: to do some long-distance running. I was determined to do six-mile runs outside the gym. I do those miles very slowly. Even though I'm strong—I can deadlift 225 pounds, which is a hefty weight for any woman—I'm not as fast on my feet as I was as a kid. And because I'm comfortable in the gym, I know I must acknowledge that, on the track, I'm a beginner as a long-distance runner.

As we think about a new fitness program, can we allow ourselves to be beginners? To do so, we need to give ourselves a break. We need to let ourselves achieve something that's really new for us by setting a modest goal, going after it, and achieving it. I need to tell myself that answers aren't always found in the gym. Sometimes answers are found inside our heads. Setting new fitness goals and sticking with them takes you beyond the physical into another realm entirely. You have to be realistic, though, about what your training goals are. Your goal can't be to look like a 20-year-old when you're actually 35, because you'll only set yourself up for failure. Set yourself up for success instead. Your goal might be: *I'm going to look like the best 35-year-old I know how to be. I have an image of the perfect 35-year-old, and that's where I'm headed. I have an image that I'm going to be better at 40 than I am at 35, and I know it can happen because I'm much better at 35 than I was at 30.*

Finding Your Strength

What you need to do now is find your strength, the strength you need to get started on an exercise routine and see it through to completion. The process involves pushing just a little bit so that you're not just going through the motions. Does that mean more weight? No. Does it mean faster or more reps? Not necessarily. It means bringing more attention to the matter at hand. How much can you feel it? How much more intently can you focus? Every time you work out, you bring with you all those other workouts you've done, and you build on them—because some days when you don't want to get up and get started, the only thing that will get you up is the memory of the fact that you were able to do it yesterday.

So where do you find your strength? You follow the exercises that are laid out in Part II, and you have faith. Why do you have faith? Maybe because you believe Montel. Maybe because you connect to the 35-year-old trainer who's not a model but who's on the cover of this book. Maybe because your friend tried the program and recommended it. Maybe because you've read this book, it makes sense, and you really believe you can make the BodyChange program work.

So you do a couple of the workouts, even if you're not so sure. And then you feel better, and you feel the muscles in your legs toning up, and you begin to see a bit of definition in your body that you never had before. You feel that your arms are stronger, and you realize after the first 21 days that you're lifting more weight—or you're lifting weights that you never lifted before. These aren't imaginary results. You'll *see* them and you'll *feel* them.

Going Outside the Comfort Zone

I've mentioned the comfort zone before, but it's essential to your success with the BodyChange program to understand what I really mean by going outside the comfort zone. It's an exercise term I use frequently, but it also has to do with your attitude toward your fitness routines and toward your life.

Your comfort zone is what you're capable of doing with no problem, where you're merely going through the motions. It's what's familiar, what's easy, what you've already done, and what you're now doing—both working out and in life. To improve yourself, to make the changes you desire in your body as well as your life, you must raise the ante and stretch beyond what feels familiar.

Every person has the desire to improve. No one wants to stay so comfortable that he or she stops growing. So choose where you want to make improvements. Do you want to be a better runner? Decrease your body fat? Have better posture? To improve, we need to edge forward into a place where we aren't so confident or capable, but where we have faith in ourselves. When we train ourselves to face obstacles, we affirm our ability to adapt to the challenge. We learn to enjoy working hard, for we know it's beyond that hard work that we improve, and see our body change.

Hard work, particularly in the form of challenging workouts, can seem scary if you haven't ever done them or it's been a long time. Yet the thought of hard work is much more frightening than the actual work itself. Break the effort down into smaller pieces and tackle it. Here's how I teach the students in my indoor cycling class to go outside their comfort zone: During what I call a climb (a period of time in which we're pedaling with enough resistance to make it difficult but manageable), I ask them to double their speed for 30 seconds. Now we're working at an intensity that we could absolutely not sustain for ten minutes, five minutes, or maybe even two minutes, but for 30 seconds we can do it. It's hard, but we can do it. That's going outside your comfort zone.

Moving beyond complacency—beyond the comfort zone—is essential in making the changes we seek. Too often we get caught up in complacency. We become so used to the status quo that we forget that inside of us is this awesome ability to change. And hard work is scary. Yet it's more frightening to remain the same. It's exciting to know we can change. There's no need to tell ourselves to get motivated when we're feeling ourselves getting stronger. We learn to embrace going beyond the comfort zone. We learn to apply the concept of stretching the limits to the rest of our lives. We learn that it takes work to build our bodies, to advance our careers, and to fortify our relationships.

ɕ ɕ ɕ

CHAPTER 5

The BodyChange Program: Let's Get Started!

The BodyChange program is a three-week jump-start into fitness. The 21-day model is a way to make exercise a part of your daily life. Twenty-one days is a measurable amount of time to commit to. After the first three weeks, you can evaluate your progress. Is the amount of weight you're lifting too easy for you? How do you know when to increase it? If you can do the required repetitions easily, you can add to the weight by a small amount. Give yourself a challenge.

When do you go from the beginner to the intermediate program? When you can complete your beginner program comfortably. One step in front of the other will take you through your journey. Each workout plan of 21 days is structured to take you from your weight workout through your aerobic workout. After each 21-day cycle, you can assess your situation. You can see, by keeping track in a workout log or diary, where you've improved. Go over your log before each workout. If the last workout was completed easily, you know that it's time to increase the weight.

Of course, there are some changes that are not so easily measured. Are you standing taller? Do you feel more alert and well rested? Progress comes in both leaps and small steps. Let the workouts pile up, and the results will come.

As for moving on to the intermediate level, some people need to build up strength to be able to do step-ups or reverse sit-ups. If an exercise is uncomfortable, choose a different variation for that body part. Each body part provides variations of exercises you can choose from. Within each program, there's plenty of room for progression without going to the next level. Before you change the exercises, you want to *own* them. Increase the weight. Focus on form. At the same time, you're putting in your minutes of aerobics and doing your basic stretches. Remember that each workout is a small victory.

What You Need to Begin the BodyChange Program

The beauty of the BodyChange program is that you don't need to belong to a fancy gym—or any gym at all—to do the workout completely and receive maximum benefit from it. You will begin to see changes in your body without having to change your venue. All you need is an area within your living space in which to perform the exercises. You will need to borrow, adapt, or buy some basic equipment in order to do the exercise routines, but these purchases do not necessarily involve a large outlay of money. If you belong to a gym, great! Most gyms have all the equipment you need (in fact, much more equipment than you'll need) to perform the BodyChange program. If you don't belong to a gym, don't worry! You can make the BodyChange program your own—anytime, anywhere. Montel travels quite a bit for his job, and he rarely misses a workout—even when he can't get to a gym.

What to Wear

Be comfortable. Don't worry about wearing tights or something revealing. Wear whatever you like. I have clients who wear clothing to show off their bodies, and then there are those who feel that they're "under construction" and are more comfortable staying covered up. You should wear something that gives you freedom to move, something that doesn't restrict full range of motion.

The one thing that is critical, however, is the right pair of shoes, which allows you to optimize your workouts. If you plan on walking or jogging for your aerobic program, purchase a shoe that will help you do so safely. Even if you're exercising at home, please don't do the routine without the right training shoes on. The proper shoe will help you in your choice of aerobic activity and your weight-training program. Go to a store where a knowledgeable sales person can help you select the appropriate shoe.

Training at Home

In order to get the maximum benefit from your BodyChange fitness routine, you'll need to set aside an area in your house or apartment in which to perform the exercises. Find a place where there's enough room for you to move, as well as store your equipment. Ideally, you should have plenty of space, but if necessary, keep your bench and weights in a corner of a room and move it to the center of the room for your workout.

The Importance of Mirrors

Working out in front of a mirror will give you visual feedback on how you're performing the exercises. You'll be able to see when you're performing a movement correctly, and associate the feeling of the correct movement with a visual image. Visualizing the proper way to perform a movement is an essential part of learning to do it right.

A mirror can be your coach. How do you look doing the exercise? Are you balanced? Are both sides of your body working evenly? How's your posture? For so many of the exercises, the mirror is your guide to the proper way to do them. Look at your body, your form, and your alignment. Chances are, the better you *look* doing it, the better you *are* doing it!

If you're training in a public gym, don't be embarrassed about working out close to the mirror. That's why there are so many mirrors in gyms—so you can see what you're doing and make sure you're doing it right!

Free Weights

You'll need to make a set of dumbbells a high priority as you plan your budget and make out your shopping list for your BodyChange program. If you've never thrown the iron around and are a true beginner to weight training, you'll want to begin with a set of 2-, 3-, 5-, and 10-pound weights for a woman; and 5-, 10-, 15-, and 20-pound weights if you're a man. You'll find that the amount of weight you can handle will increase quite quickly. As you become stronger, your muscles adapt and require more of a challenge. So when you're buying free weights, be sure you get several different weights at the same time. You'll need them sooner than you think.

The Swiss Ball

Two years ago at my gym, there wasn't a Swiss ball (also called a gym ball or exercise ball) to be had. Now they're everywhere you look. Almost every gym has a variety of exercise balls. You can find people lying, kneeling, sitting or even standing on them. Ball training can be incorporated into every workout routine. Swiss balls help you improve your balance, coordination, and body awareness. The Swiss ball is designed to hold an adult's body size and weight.

In any case, a Swiss ball is a good purchase because once you become proficient at doing abdominal exercises on your floor mat, you'll want to vary your routine. Attempting to perform crunches on a Swiss ball the first time is an exhilarating experience: You think you know how to do them, but you've never done them like this—leaning back against a big, bright cushion of a ball. Not only does your body face a balance challenge as you perform the crunch, but now your abs can move through a greater range of motion than they do when you're just lying flat on the floor. There's more resistance—as well as more fun—when doing crunches on a Swiss ball.

A variety of exercises can be used with the Swiss ball. Anything you do while sitting on a bench can be done sitting on a Swiss ball. The difference is that a Swiss ball is unstable; therefore, your body has to be stable. Once you master a standing lateral raise, for instance, try doing it on a Swiss ball. Give your body a riddle to solve.

The Incline Bench

In order to perform certain free-weight and functional exercises, you'll need an adjustable incline bench. It must be heavy enough to support your weight without scooting away as you do push-ups on it or step up onto it. An adjustable incline bench is a smart purchase to make because you can do a variety of exercises on it. You can sit on it or lie back on it. You can also work at various inclines to challenge your muscles in different ways

The Heart-Rate Monitor

The heart-rate monitor is one of the most useful devices in the fitness world. Everyone—from the beginner to the elite athlete—can benefit from wearing one. You can use it for both your aerobic workout and your interval training, so I highly recommend that you use one.

A wireless heart-rate monitor, the kind you use in sports training, consists of a wrist receiver that looks like a watch, and a chest strap with a transmitter that picks up your heart rate and sends it to the receiver. The wrist receiver often has a watch and a stopwatch feature, although you don't need it to measure your heart rate. The most important thing is to be able to see the numbers clearly while you're exercising. You don't need a heart-rate monitor with a lot of fancy bells and whistles. Start out with the basic model, and as you learn how to use it, decide how much fancier you need to get. (Later in this book, when I discuss the aerobic part of your workout routine, I'll give you additional information about these monitors.)

Don't be put off by the notion of wearing a heart-rate monitor. Once you learn how to use it, your aerobic workouts will become more interesting as you monitor your progress.

The Medicine Ball

A medicine ball looks like a large soccer ball, but comes in a variety of weights and is used to vary exercise routines. Medicine balls are useful when performing core and functional exercises. Montel uses the medicine ball to increase the resistance he feels while performing reverse sit-ups, thereby providing more of a challenge to his abdominal muscles.

A medicine ball is a beneficial piece of equipment to own if you have the space to store it and can afford to buy one.

Your Favorite Music

Music is one the greatest wonders of the world and can really help you during your workouts. Although some people are distracted by music, if it's your personal stereo you're listening to with your own choice of music, that can make all the difference—as it can help you dial in to whatever you're feeling at the moment.

I love to listen to my favorite music while I train. I start my workout as soon as I put the mini headphones on. I know people who listen to opera, and I know those who listen to dance music. I usually keep a variety of tapes in my locker, ranging from show tunes to gospel.

Put on whatever moves you. Then move!

Toss the Scale

Get rid of it! Montel is the biggest proponent of tossing the scale. Measure your progress in the mirror, or by how your clothes fit. Muscle is much denser than fat and weighs more. An average man can gain five pounds while losing at least an inch in his waistline in 21 days. A woman can easily lose a dress size. Getting on a scale can sabotage you faster than anything else. A little salt can cause five pounds of water retention and, again, undermine your motivation. So at least for the first 21-day program, don't weigh yourself.

℣ ℣ ℣

CHAPTER 6

The Importance
of Functional Exercise

The Basic Exercises That Yield Results

Montel: *One of the things I started doing with Wini is more free-weight exercises. Of course they're harder, yet they're really effective when doing squats, one-arm rows, and lateral raises. I've tried every machine out there, but there's nothing comparable to throwing those weights around—feeling strong and working hard. That's the best way to train—hard!*

• • •

In the gym, we need to work our muscles the way they're meant to be used—*together*. Standing, lunging, bending, squatting—these movements are designed to challenge your muscles to work together while keeping your posture perfect and your awareness high. I said this earlier, but I'm going to review it again quickly because the functional exercises are the basis of BodyChange. In real life, we aren't asked to sit on a machine and push, yet we're often called upon to walk up the stairs, open windows, and carry packages. In what real-life situation would you sit on a machine and extend your knees? We need to learn to use all our muscles *together*. Think about crouching down to greet a child—a complex combination of muscles is working there.

I'm not saying that machines don't have their place in an exercise program—variety is the spice of life. However, the core of your program—even if you do have access to machines—should be free-weight exercises. Push-ups, squats, and lunges require movement and balance. We present our body with an additional puzzle to which it must find a solution. We need to use our bodies fully, to balance and coordinate and *move.*

The movements that require you to balance and guide your body weight through a range of motion are what I call **functional exercises.** If you perform a leg press on an exercise machine, it's certainly a challenge. Yet if you perform a squat instead, it's a much greater challenge. To perform a squat, you'll not only develop strength in all the muscle groups of your legs, but also balance and coordination. A squat makes demands on your whole body that a leg press doesn't. By employing your upper body and your abdominals in addition to your entire lower body, you're putting in the same time that you would on the machine, but you're getting back so much more.

Functional exercises provide strength in motion. But what good is strength if it can't be used in our day-to-day lives?

Machines vs. Free Weights

Montel: *I have access to a lot of different equipment. I prefer a full set of dumbbells, a bench, and an hour. Give me that, and I have my workout set.*

• • •

If you're strapped into a machine, your body doesn't learn to master the complex movements that combine more than one muscle group—which are necessary to produce any movement in life outside the gym.

Another reason why free weights are preferable to machines has to do with balanced strength. If one side of your body is stronger than the other, you'll never find that out by using machines. Let's say that your right leg is stronger than your left.

You won't be able to determine that when you use some machines; therefore, you won't be able to correct the problem. Doing a walking lunge goes a long way to even up the sides.

Another example is this: You may be able to press 100 pounds on a chest machine, but is that weight evenly distributed, or are you pressing more with your stronger side? If you use two 50-pound dumbbells, one in each hand, the difference will be apparent. You can then work to correct the imbalance, either by doing extra reps with the weaker side, or by increasing the weight slightly on that side and performing the same number of reps until you strengthen it.

Another reason I prefer free weights is that machines are built for the average person . . . and I have yet to meet the average person. (If I did meet the average person and pointed out how average he was, he might well be within his rights to take his average-size hand and hit me over the head for insulting his average-size ego!) Most of the female athletes I train have trouble fitting into the machines that were developed for the so-called average-size man. Machines are adjustable to some extent, but with free weights, each human body gets maximum return for each amount of effort that's put forth—that is, nothing is wasted, as it can be with man-made machines.

Machines are certainly a great addition to an exercise program, but the most efficient use of your time and energy will be made by using your own body weight and free weights to do most of the work.

$$\mathcal{L} \quad \mathcal{L} \quad \mathcal{L}$$

CHAPTER 7

Smart Aerobics

What Is Aerobic Exercise?

Aerobics refers to any activity that uses oxygen. In a fitness program, aerobic exercise refers to a sustained activity such as cycling, jogging, or swimming that elevates your heart rate over a sustained period of time. It should get you breathing deeply yet not leave you short of breath.

Montel is passionate about snowboarding, which he does just as soon as the snow falls on the slopes. When he can't snowboard, he hits the treadmill. Choose something that *you* can do, and plan to keep doing it for at least 20 minutes. If you have to start with a little less time, that's fine. It's important that you just begin.

So let's get moving! The most important muscle—yes, even more important than defined abdominals and buff biceps—is the heart. No one dies from weak biceps. It's important to strengthen our hearts so we can live our lives to the fullest.

My client Linda was very comfortable with her aerobic exercise when she came to me—in fact, she was a bit *too* comfortable. She would sit on the bike for 30 minutes, three days a week. She believed she was burning more fat by exercising at a lower intensity, so she would read the paper, chat on her cell phone, and do everything she could to avoid breaking a sweat. The first thing I did was shatter the fat-burning myth.

Some people think that the longer they can last on an aerobic machine, the better a workout they get and the more fat they're burning. But losing weight through exercise depends on the number of calories you burn compared to the number you ingest. It's true that the percentage of fat burned by your body is higher when you do a lower-intensity workout than when you do one of a higher intensity, but the total number of calories expended is always greater at a higher intensity. You burn more calories when you exercise more intensely, even though the percentage of calories your body uses comes from carbohydrate rather than fat metabolism.

There are three components of aerobic activity:

1. **Frequency**—How many times each week you exercise.

2. **Duration**—The length of each exercise period. Once you achieve your target heart rate, try to sustain your aerobic activity for at least 20 minutes.

3. **Intensity**—How hard you're working. If you don't have a heart-rate monitor, a good way to estimate how hard you're working is to use the rate of perceived exertion. This refers to intensity levels, with level 1 being your body at rest, reading, or standing in line; and level 10 being a full sprint up a steep hill with maximum effort. Depending upon your goals and fitness level, you generally want to keep your aerobic workout between 5 (walking at a moderate pace) and 8 (moderate running).

Finding the Right Activity for You

As I mentioned previously, Montel likes snowboarding whenever he can, or walking briskly on the treadmill when he's in the gym. I love teaching my Spinning™ classes on the weekends and doing my own aerobics on the cardio equipment in the gym. Some of my other clients have their own preferences: Janice runs in Central

Park, Julie enjoys listening to audio books on the elliptical trainer, Alice goes to a local pool to swim, and Mindy jumps rope.

What can *you* do? Here are some suggestions:

Stationary Bike

An upright stationary bike can be found in almost every gym. It's also a practical piece of equipment to have at home, since it's not as expensive or space-consuming as a treadmill. It's easy to use, and you don't have to worry about being distracted by traffic lights and rollerbladers.

Recumbent Bike

A recumbent bike is a stationary bike that gives you low back support. Many beginners or those with lower back problems find exercising on a recumbent bike more comfortable than using an upright stationary bike because your legs are in front of your hips, thus taking pressure off the back.

Elliptical Trainer

An elliptical trainer keeps you upright in a moving position, yet is easier on the joints than running or jogging. Elliptical trainers move you in an elliptical movement, simulating the effects of running without the impact on the joints.

Stair Stepper

This machine keeps you moving without impact as well. It simulates walking up stairs, or a climbing motion. Be sure not to lean into the machine; and try to take big, natural steps.

Treadmill

You can walk, jog, or run on a treadmill. It's fine if you alternate walking and jogging. This is Montel's favorite way to get in his aerobics. You can vary the speed and the incline on a treadmill as well.

Training Smarter with a Heart-Rate Monitor

Heart-rate monitors are a window into the body. Everyone, from the beginner to the elite athlete, can benefit from them.

Using a heart-rate monitor can help you answer the following questions:

- What is my heart rate?
- How can I tell if my aerobic program is working?
- How can I change my approach when I want to run a marathon instead of my usual five miles?
- How will I know when I need to take it easy?
- How will I know if I've improved my aerobic conditioning enough to do a 50-mile bike ride?

With weight training, I can look at a person's body and tell which weights and at what intensity they need to redesign their body's shape. I take into account the person's current fitness level, the amount of time they have per week to train, and their short- and long-term goals. I can measure a person's strength and flexibility. But a heart-rate monitor is the only way to measure what's going on in someone's heart.

Heart-rate monitors keep you on track. It's like having a speedometer on your body. It measures your heart rate so you can pace yourself. It tells you if you're working too hard or taking it too easy. A heart-rate monitor lets you know when you can push a little more or need to take the intensity down a notch.

A common situation I see in the gym is people who are walking along on their treadmill, speaking on their cell phones or even reading the paper. Some people look like they're taking it so easy that they could fall asleep! Again, everything depends on what their goal is, but if it's to strengthen their heart, they probably have to work a bit harder than the leisurely pace they appear to be taking.

However, right next to this type of person could be someone who's holding on for dear life to the treadmill. This individual is pushing so hard that they look like they're going to keel over! Somewhere in between these two lies the correct intensity, and it can be found using a heart-rate monitor. Using one actually makes doing aerobics much easier and a whole lot more interesting and enjoyable.

Heart-rate monitors have two parts: (1) The strap has a sensor in it that picks up your heartbeat and transmits it to a separate piece that looks like a wristwatch; and (2) the watch displays your heart rate. There are different functions and features in the various heart-rate monitors that are available, but the most important thing is that you can see the numbers clearly.

My client Laura always used the treadmill, but it bored her since she never felt like she could really work up a sweat. Using the heart-rate monitor, she finally started training at the right intensity. It was a bit of a challenge, yet not so hard that she couldn't sustain it. She learned that at her target heart rate, she could push herself intensely for 30 minutes and work up a good sweat. All she had to do was find that target heart rate and stay there.

Figuring Your Resting, Maximum, and Target Heart Rates

Making sure you're working at your *target* heart rate, which is 65 to 85 percent of your *maximum* heart rate, is essential to working with a heart-rate monitor. A beginner should build a base by working at 65 percent. Advanced exercisers can spend more time in the 75 percent range.

Throughout the book, I'll answer some frequently asked questions such as the following:

What is resting heart rate?

Resting heart rate can be an indicator of your basic fitness level. The more conditioned the body, the less effort and fewer beats per minute it takes your heart to pump blood throughout your body. You can lower your resting heart rate by becoming more aerobically fit.

To determine your resting heart rate, measure your heart rate first thing in the morning before you get out of bed. Do it for five mornings in a row, and then average the readings.

How do I figure out my maximum heart rate?

You can have it tested, use predicted maximum heart rate (MAX HR) formulas, or self-administer a sub-max test. The accurate assessment of your MAX HR is crucial to individualizing your training. The most accurate MAX HR tests are given in a lab. We can do a guesstimate of our max and adjust it by our rate of perceived exertion. You can predict your maximum heart rate by using two different formulas: *age-predicted,* or the *Karvonen* formula.

Age-predicted estimate:

- 220 minus age for men equals maximum heart rate
- 226 minus age for women equals maximum heart rate

The age-adjusted formula can be off by as much as ten beats. That's a lot when you're trying to figure out your zones. Not every 25- or 35- or 45-year-old woman is the same, so the formula was based on the theory that max heart rate declines with age. If you train aerobically, your heart rate doesn't necessarily decline with age; therefore, the age-predicted formula cannot apply. The formula provides an estimate— a number to keep in mind—yet you still need to adjust the number by as much as ten beats.

The Karvonen formula is more indicative of your true training zones because it takes your resting heart rate into the equation:

220 – age – resting heart x __ % of training + resting heart rate

For example:

A fit 40-year-old wants to know what her 80% training zone is.
She has a resting heart rate of 68.

220 – 40 = 180 – 68 = 112 x .80 + 68 = 157

She would work out around 157 beats per minute for a very intense workout.

How do I figure out my target heart rate?

Once you have your maximum heart rate number, you can figure your target heart rate number by multiplying your maximum heart rate by 65 percent for beginners. Once you build an aerobic base, you can work at a higher percentage. You should be able to sustain the intensity level for at least 20 minutes.

What about my recovery heart rate?

One of the best indicators of fitness is the ability to recover quickly by returning to your working recovery rate following training. Record your heart rate at one, two, and five minutes following exercise. Over time and with training, you'll see a more rapid return to its pre-exercise rate. The stronger you are, the faster you'll recover.

What heart rate should I look for in my aerobic exercise?

The answer goes back to the original questions:

- What are your goals?
- What is your starting point?
- How long have you been working out?
- Is this your first aerobic conditioning session this week, or your fourth?
- Did you work out hard yesterday?
- How long a workout do you want to do?

Take Lisa, for example. Her maximum heart rate for running is 198. She's been training on the treadmill for nine months and wants to improve her athletic performance. She brought her twin sister, Linda, with her, who has the same maximum heart rate but is training for the marathon and wants a less intense aerobic workout (but one she can sustain for a longer period of time).

If they train at different intensity levels, they'll look for different target heart-rate levels.

Linda, the marathoner, wants to run for a long duration. She'll use the heart-rate monitor to keep her intensity around 65 percent. Lisa, who wants to improve her general fitness level, will train at a higher intensity—around 75.

ℒ ℒ ℒ

CHAPTER 8

The Basics

The Importance of a Warm-Up

Before you get to the exercises, you have to warm up. If you're at a gym, hop on your favorite aerobic machine for 15 minutes. If you're working out at home, take a light jog or a brisk walk. Just as you need to slowly adapt to the exercises over time, you also need to slowly ease into each daily workout. A warm-up gets you ready for your workout—both mentally and physically.

A warm-up is the time to gather your thoughts, to go over in your mind what you want to accomplish in the daily workout. You can recall the workouts you've done to lead you to this point, and you can focus on the workout you're doing today that will bring you closer to your goal. The extra few minutes are really worth it. The time you spend with yourself is the best investment you can make.

Some of my clients work out first thing in the morning, while others rush to the gym straight from the office. Either way, the warm-up is important. Montel prefers to train early in the morning, and he knows that the first few minutes of the workout are very important—to both center himself and to warm up his muscles for more vigorous movement.

Sometimes the warm-up can be an opportunity to *wake* up. Breaking into a light sweat can get you in the groove of working hard. When the last thing you want to do is go to the gym after a hard day's work, a few minutes on the bike can help you remember how much you enjoy your training time.

What about sets and reps?

A **rep** or a **repetition** is a single movement of an exercise. To squat once is one repetition. A **set** is a *group* of repetitions; for example, ten repetitions of a squat is one set of ten. Most of the weight exercises in the BodyChange program specify 12 reps. What that means is that if you can't do at least 12, the weight needs to be lighter. On the other hand, if you can do more than 15 comfortably, the weight is too light and it's time to increase it so that 10 reps are again a challenge for you.

Listen to your body first. If in doubt, use a lighter weight that you can execute more reps on until you're more confident about your form.

The Order of the Exercises

In the BodyChange program, we always work the larger muscle groups (such as the chest and back) first. We don't want to fatigue the smaller muscle groups (such as the triceps and biceps) before we fatigue the larger ones. Since we use the biceps in our back exercises, we need to have the biceps strong to help us challenge the back. We need to exercise in the right order so we can challenge our muscle groups fully. If we tire the weak parts, we won't get through the workout. We're only as strong as out weakest link.

How much weight do I start with?

You need to choose your starting weight with a guesstimate. You're much better off beginning with a slightly lighter weight than you think you need. If you can easily do 10 repetitions, yet cannot do 15 repetitions in good form, you've found a good starting weight for that exercise.

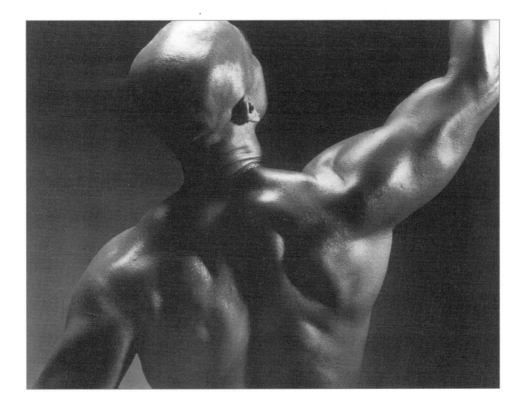

Sticking Points

Each free-weight exercise has a **sticking point,** the point at which it's the most difficult. The bottom of a bicep curl or the full bend of a squat—those are the points at which the exercise becomes most difficult and are the ones we must pay more attention to. The sticking point is the part we're looking for, the point that we need to push through. Some parts of an exercise are always easier, but the difficult points are the ones we need to embrace.

Rest Between Sets

How long should you rest between sets? That question can be answered with another question: *What are your goals?* When Montel trains really heavily, we rest longer between sets. A good rule of thumb is to rest from 30 seconds to one minute for the basic program.

Breathing

Exhale on effort (of course it's all effort). Exhale as you lift the weight. Inhale as you lower the weight. Don't think too hard about breathing, because if you do, you may wind up holding your breath. Don't overanalyze your breathing to the point where you're hyperventilating. Just remember that the general rule of thumb in training is to *exhale on effort.* It should happen naturally.

Good Pain vs. Bad Pain

Montel: *There's a simple rule that Wini and I follow in the gym: We figure out if it's good pain or bad pain.*

Nothing you do when performing a workout should ever be painful. Your muscles and your entire body simply need to feel *challenged*—that's what we call good pain. Bad pain is what you feel in a joint or tendon. You don't ever want to fatigue a body part to the point that it feels that kind of pain, because that's when you could get injured. If you're not sure if you can do something, use no weight or a smaller range of motion to start.

Challenging your muscles will cause lactic acid to build up in them, which produces the burning sensation you sometimes feel when you exercise intensely. Training hard *will* make your muscles feel fatigued, but it should never feel like a jolting or sharp pain.

Good pain truly isn't pain—it just means you're giving your body a challenge. It will adapt by getting stronger. Bad pain means *stop,* check what you're doing, lighten the weight, or do something else. Listen to your body. *This is your ride.*

Montel said this earlier, but it's important so I'm going to repeat it: *You're going to be sore!* This is good pain. But the only way to push through this is to *move!* The soreness is caused by the lactic acid buildup in your muscles. The only way to push this out is to keep the blood pumping through them. If you're really too sore to do your BodyChange routine, at least take a brisk walk. Get yourself moving.

℮ ℮ ℮

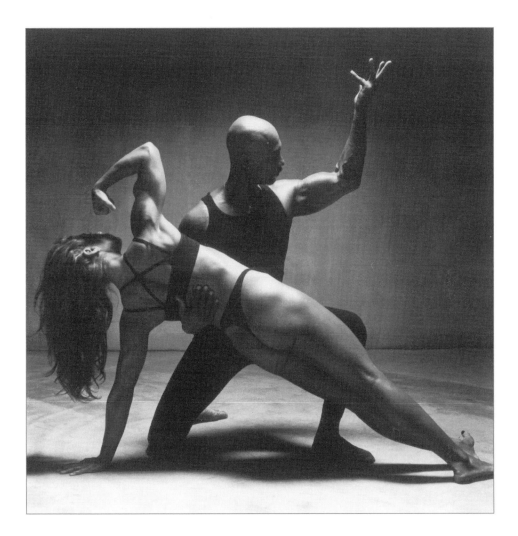

PART II

• The Exercises •

CHAPTER 9

LowerBodyChange

All of the following exercises are **functional exercises,** large movements that integrate many muscle groups. Like all real-life movements that are performed every day, your muscles learn to work together to meet the challenge. Your body adapts to the challenge by getting stronger. Adapting to the challenge, then surpassing it, is what BodyChange is all about.

The primary muscle groups targeted in the following exercises are:

Gluteals: The muscles of the buttocks, which you can feel when you extend your hip.

Hamstrings: The muscles at the back of the upper leg. They're the muscles that work when you bend your knee.

Quadriceps: The muscles of the upper front leg. They're flexed when you extend your knee to straighten your leg.

Abductors: The muscles on the side of the leg. They're used when you lift your leg to the side.

Adductors: The muscles of the inner thigh. They're used when you move your leg across your body.

Calves: The muscles of the back of the lower legs.

BODYCHANGE TIPS
FOR TRAINING
YOUR LOWER BODY

1. Always set up your body in the starting position, which is **neutral stance.** Neutral stance means that you're standing in correct alignment. Keep your knees soft (not locked into place), your hips square, your shoulders even, and your neck elongated. Line up your joints with your shoulders in line with your hips, your knees in line with your hips, and your ankles in line with your knees.

2. Maintain a constant drawing-in and lifting of the abdominals. It's not about holding your breath; it's about holding your posture.

3. Imagine your bones evenly stacked one on top of the other, with a string attached to the top of your head that's keeping you aligned and balanced.

4. As you focus on the quality of each rep, try to feel the muscles working to move you. The goal is not *how many* reps you can do, but *how few* you can do.

5. Move at a slow pace. Descend and then ascend with purpose.

6. Start slowly. In mastering these movements, be prepared to be a beginner. You may not feel the exercise at first, but practice being aware of the feeling of the movement. With practice, the mind gets stronger, along with the muscles.

7. Learn to embrace the sticking points, because that's where your body learns to adapt to the challenge. *The hard part of the exercise is precisely the part you need to do.*

SQUAT

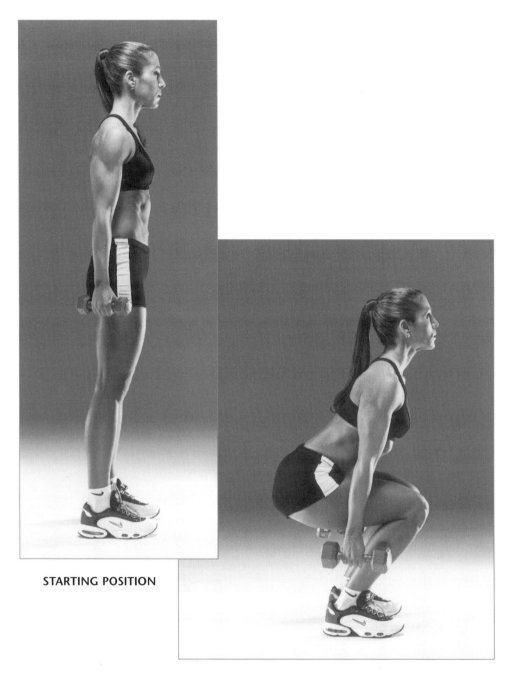

STARTING POSITION

MOVEMENT

SQUAT

STARTING POSITION:

- Stand in neutral stance.
- Keep your feet hip-width apart.
- Look straight ahead, with your abdominals drawn in and your rib cage lifted.
- Bend your knees a bit.
- Point your toes outward slightly.

MOVEMENT:

- Bend your knees (as if you're taking a seat) until your thighs are parallel to the floor and your knees are in line with your hips.
- Keep your body weight toward your heels, with your heels touching the floor at all times and your chest up.
- Push back up to a starting position by lengthening your legs in one fluid movement.

TRAINING TIPS:

- Keep abdominals in. Remember: Don't hold your breath; hold your posture.
- Keep your back in a neutral position. Try not to bend at the waist.
- Lengthen your legs without locking your knees.
- Don't go past the parallel hip position (in relation to the floor) on the descent.
- Keep your chin lifted.
- Try to keep your heels on the ground. If you can't, place a half-inch block under your heels.
- As you sit into the squat, visualize sitting on a chair.

• • •

BEGINNER DUMBBELL SQUAT
LEANING AGAINST A SWISS BALL

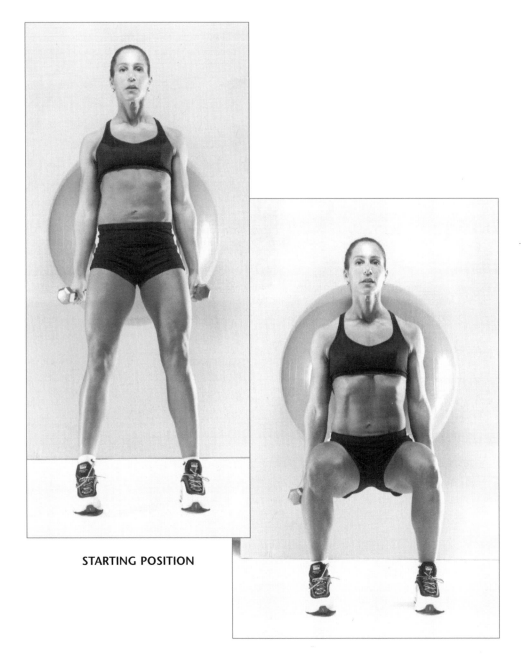

STARTING POSITION

MOVEMENT

BEGINNER DUMBBELL SQUAT LEANING AGAINST A SWISS BALL

STARTING POSITION:

- Place the Swiss ball against a wall at lower back level, and lean against it.
- Stand with your feet hip-width apart, with the dumbbells in your hands at your sides.

MOVEMENT:

- Keeping your chest up, bend your knees until your thighs are parallel to the floor.
- Push back up to a starting position.

REMEMBER:

- Keep your abdominals tucked in during the entire movement.
- Look up slightly as you perform the movement.
- Keep your heels on the ground.

The Swiss ball provides back support that allows you to go deeper than you might in a traditional dumbbell squat. It also keeps you upright so your focus can remain on your thighs. The dumbbells provide additional resistance and challenge to the upper body.

BODYCHANGE BONUS:

For variation, use a wider stance with your feet turned out. This position challenges your adductors (inner thighs) a bit more.

BODYCHANGE BLAST:

For the last set, do a drop set. Do 12 repetitions with light dumbbells in your hands, then immediately put them down and do 12 to 15 more without any additional weight.

Tip: *Look in the mirror.*

One of my clients, Alicia, age 37, was very resistant to doing squats. She had tried them at home while watching exercise videos and always found that her ankles wobbled and she leaned over too much. She couldn't seem to find her balance, and she felt silly because the exercise looked so simple to perform.

Instead of squatting in front of her TV, I taught her how to squat in front of a mirror. By doing so while performing this "simple" exercise, Alicia developed a sense of how she looked in relation to how she felt, as well as where she was in relation to the floor.

• • •

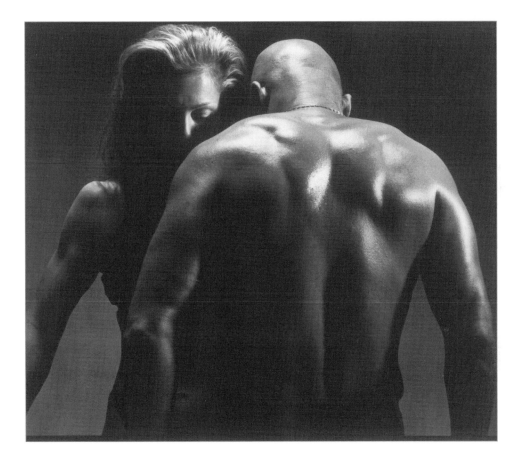

WALKING LUNGE

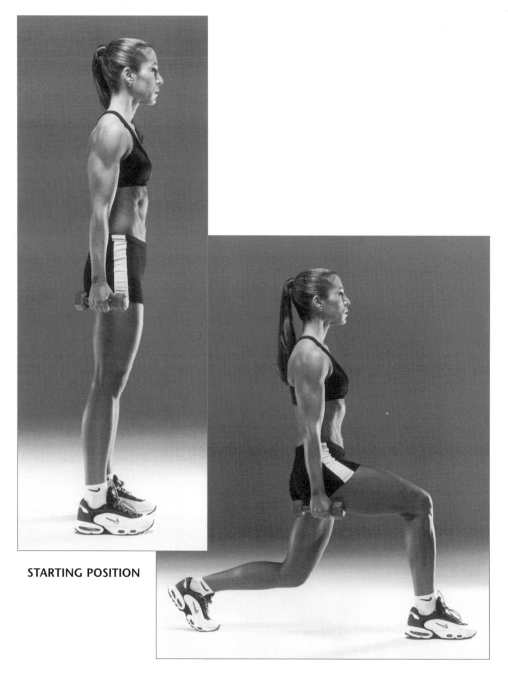

STARTING POSITION

MOVEMENT

WALKING LUNGE

Lunges are difficult to do, yet we need a challenge, and our body will adapt to the challenge by becoming stronger.

Lunges challenge the muscles of our lower body, shaping them while we learn to increase our power. Lunges teach us how to move forward in perfect form. They are important functional exercises and can be done anywhere: on the beach or down a hotel corridor if necessary.

STARTING POSITION:

- Stand tall in neutral stance.
- Keep your abdominals tucked in, with your shoulders under your hips and your knees relaxed.
- Hold a light dumbbell in each hand.

MOVEMENT:

- Take a large step forward, leading with the heel until your front ankle and knee are in a straight line.
- Push your front heel into the floor, then pause as you recheck your alignment
- Lift yourself up and transfer your weight forward onto the opposite leg.
- Walk across the room until you've completed 10 to 16 steps.

TRAINING TIPS:

- Focus on your posture, and keep your shoulders aligned with your hips.
- Dig your front heel into the floor to feel your glutes.
- Do not bend at the waist. Keep your spine long, as if there's a string attached to the top of your head pulling you up to the ceiling.

• • •

STEP-UPS

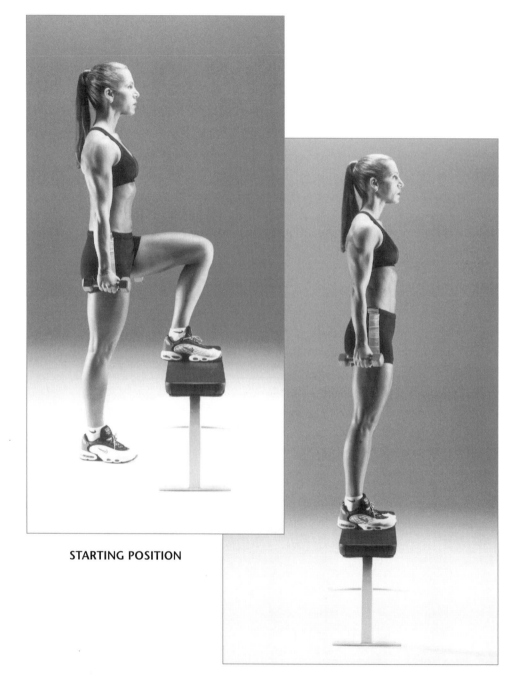

STARTING POSITION

MOVEMENT

STEP-UPS

Step-ups are a true butt-blaster exercise. To work your butt off, literally, you need to do a true extension of the hip. Think of how it looks when you push back through your hip to straighten your leg. The step-up is the same movement, with the additional challenge of moving your body through space.

STARTING POSITION:

- Stand in neutral stance in front of a bench at or slightly above knee level.
- Put your hands on your waist for balance to start.

Note: This movement is easier to perform if you can look straight ahead into a mirror.

MOVEMENT:

- Place one foot on the bench. With your knee and ankle in a straight line, step up onto it.
- Visualize pulling yourself up with the muscles of your glutes and hamstrings. Keep your hips under your shoulders and your abdominals tucked in.
- Repeat on the same leg before switching to your other leg.

REMEMBER:

- Keep your hips and shoulders squared.
- Be sure your ankle and knee are in a straight line as you step up onto the bench.
- Dig your heel into the bench as you raise your body up.
- Keep your arms close to your body during this exercise.
- Be sure to keep your spine elongated, with no bend in the waist, as you lift yourself up.

• • •

STANDING CALF RAISE

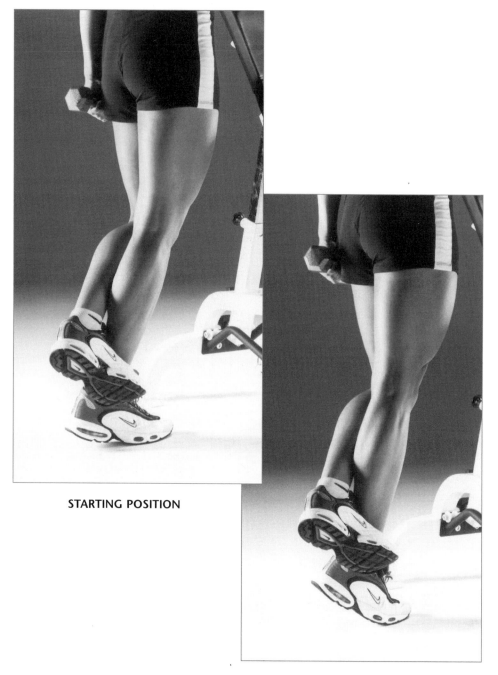

STARTING POSITION

MOVEMENT

STANDING CALF RAISE

The muscles of the lower leg include the gastrocnemius and the soleus. The gastrocnemius flexes when you raise yourself onto the ball of your foot. The soleus works when your knee is bent and you raise your heel.

STARTING POSITION:

- Stand on your right foot.
- Wrap your left foot behind your right ankle.
- Place your left hand on the wall for balance if necessary.

MOVEMENT:

- Raise your right foot up onto the ball of your foot.
- Pause for a moment at the top of the movement, and squeeze your calf like a ball before lowering your foot to the ground.

BODYCHANGE BONUS:

When this movement becomes easy, hold a light dumbbell in the opposite hand of the calf you're raising. Increase the weight to add to the intensity of this movement.

Option: *If you can do this movement on a block of wood or a platform, it lets you go through a full range of motion.*

• • •

CHAPTER 10

UpperBodyChange
Chest

Developed chest muscles are great for everyone—both women and men. It's wonderful to be strong enough to push with the powerful muscles of the chest.

The chest muscles are the pectoralis major and pectoralis minor, which are used when we press our arms or cross them in front of our bodies. These muscles assist us in pushing and throwing, and give us a feeling of strength when they're trained properly.

• • •

PUSH-UPS: BEGINNER VERSION

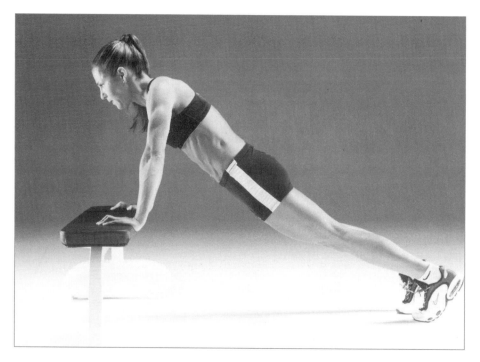

STARTING POSITION

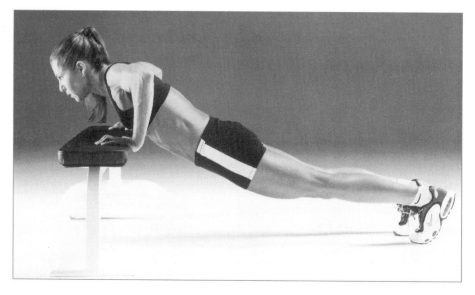

MOVEMENT

PUSH-UPS

Push-ups intimidate people, but they shouldn't. As with any exercise, the more you practice them, the better you'll do them. Give yourself a learning curve—if you've never done a push-up before, just practice holding the start position.

Push-ups are what I call a great bang-for-your-buck exercise. In addition to challenging the chest, shoulders, and triceps, push-ups require balance and coordination. *Unlike other upper-body exercises where we're moving weights through space, with push-ups we're moving ourselves.*

Beginner Version: Push-Ups on a Bench

STARTING POSITION:

- With your feet on the floor and your body perpendicular to the bench, point your hands forward on top of the bench, with your arms slightly wider than your shoulders.
- Align your body so that it's straight—from your head through your back to your ankles—with no bend at the hips.
- Elongate your neck, and look beyond the bench toward the floor so that your head remains aligned during the movement and your back remains neutral.
- Keep your shoulders in line with your hips, and your hips in line with your feet.
- Make sure your abdominals are drawn in.

MOVEMENT:

- Move your lower chest toward the bench while maintaining a straight line with your body.

- Keep this movement controlled as your chest reaches, and then lightly touches, the bench.
- Push your body up to a starting position.

REMEMBER:

- Think of your body as one long unit, with no break at the waist or hips.
- As you lower your chest toward the bench, think about stretching the muscles in your chest as if you're stretching a rubber band.
- As you push your body up off the bench, think about pushing the bench away from you into the floor and flexing your chest muscles.

Intermediate Version: Push-Ups on the Floor

STARTING POSITION:

- Place your hands on the floor under your shoulders, with your arms extended and at a slightly wider distance than your shoulders.
- Align your body so that it's straight from your head through your back to your ankles, with no bend at the hips.
- Elongate your neck and look slightly ahead.
- Keep your back straight, with your shoulders in line with your hips, and your hips in line with your feet.
- Draw in your abs so there's no bend at your hips.

MOVEMENT:

- Keeping your shoulders pressed down, lower your chest to the floor.
- Maintain a straight line with your body as you do so.
- Look ahead slightly so that your neck remains long.
- When your chest touches the floor, push your body back up with power.

PUSH-UPS: INTERMEDIATE VERSION

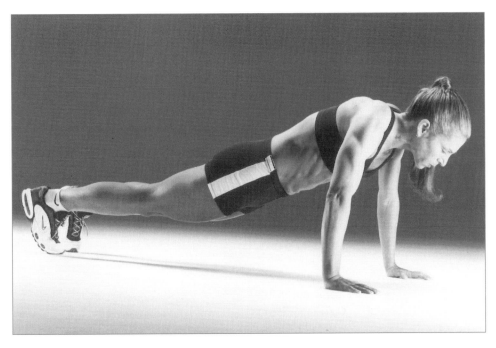

STARTING POSITION

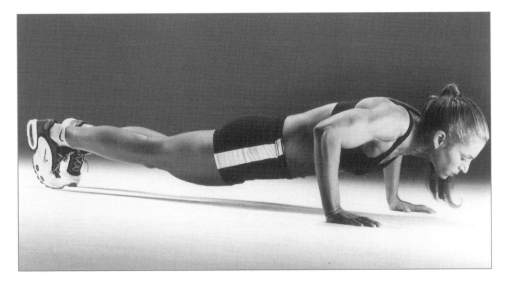

MOVEMENT

BodyChange BONUS:

To make this exercise even more of a challenge, elevate your feet on a small board.

BodyChange CHALLENGE:

Add a bit more challenge to your push-up routine by placing a small medicine ball between your knees. Not only does the weight of the ball add more resistance to your muscles, it helps you connect to your abdominals and keeps them drawn in.

Advanced Push-Ups on a Swiss Ball

Push-ups using a Swiss ball provide an additional challenge to your upper body. With your legs raised up on the big, round ball, you must not only use your chest, shoulders, and triceps, but you must also maintain your balance on an unstable surface. Your abdominals are super-challenged to keep your body stable.

STARTING POSITION:

- Place your hands on the floor under your shoulders, with your arms slightly wider than your shoulders.
- Place your feet on the Swiss ball instead of the ground.
- Align your body so that it's straight—from your head through your back to your ankles.
- Elongate your neck so that your head remains aligned, with your back straight and no bend at the waist.
- Keep your shoulders in line with your hips, and your hips in line with your feet.
- Draw in your abdominals, with no bend at the hip.

PUSH-UPS: ADVANCED VERSION

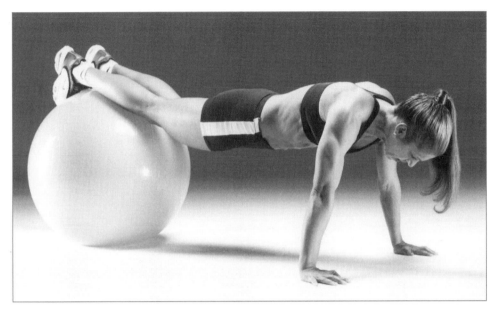

STARTING POSITION

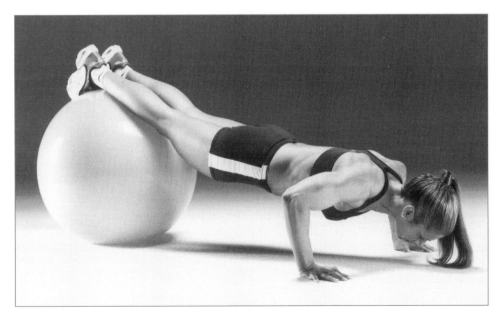

MOVEMENT

MOVEMENT:

- Hold the starting position for a few seconds to ensure that you're balanced.
- Keeping your shoulders pressed down, lower your chest toward the floor with your arms, and maintain a straight line with your body.
- Keep looking ahead as your chest lowers toward the floor, then push the floor away to raise your body.

• • •

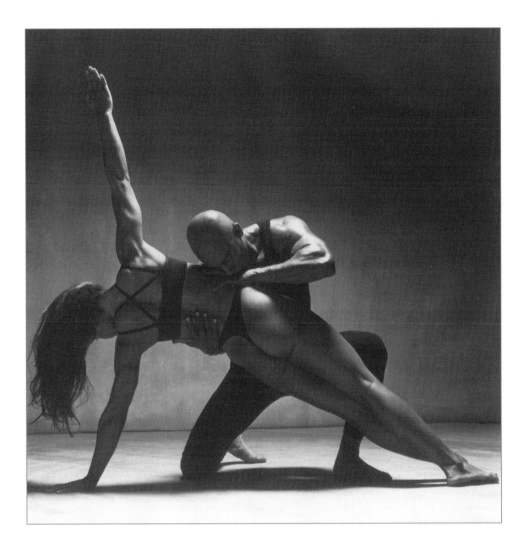

INCLINE DUMBBELL PRESS

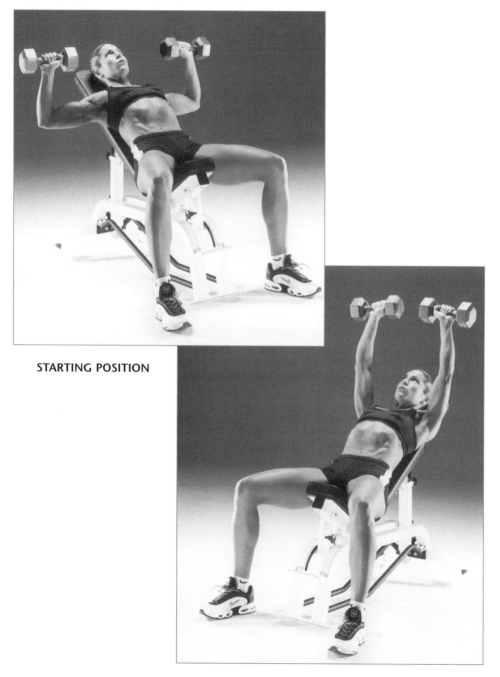

STARTING POSITION

MOVEMENT

INCLINE DUMBBELL PRESS

This exercise focuses on the upper section of your chest, while also challenging your deltoids and triceps.

STARTING POSITION:

- Lie on the bench with your feet flat on the floor.
- Grab two dumbbells, and lean back until your back is neutral against the bench, not arched.
- Your elbows should be slightly below the level of your shoulders. The dumbbells should be in line with your elbows.

MOVEMENT:

- Keeping your palms facing front, press the dumbbells up and together directly over the upper chest, forming a triangle with your arms.
- Slowly bend your arms, and lower the dumbbells until they're slightly below the level of your chest. You should feel a slight stretch in your chest.

REMEMBER:

- Keep your shoulders down.
- Lengthen your arms without locking out your elbows.
- Press your shoulders down toward the floor as you use your chest muscles to lift the weight.
- Never arch your back. Keep it neutral against the bench at all times.
- Keep your abs drawn in at all times throughout the movement.

- Dumbbells are a great way to work both sides of your body independently of each other. Unlike the movements you perform on machines, which allow your stronger side to do all the work, dumbbells challenge both sides of your body, forcing the weaker side to work harder to balance the stronger side's effort.

• • •

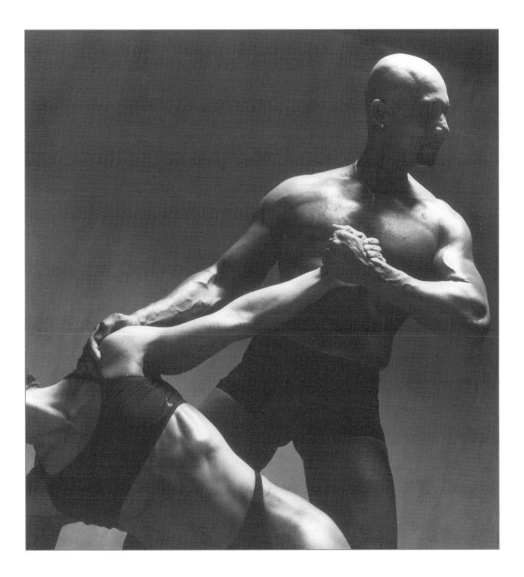

ONE-ARM DUMBBELL PRESS

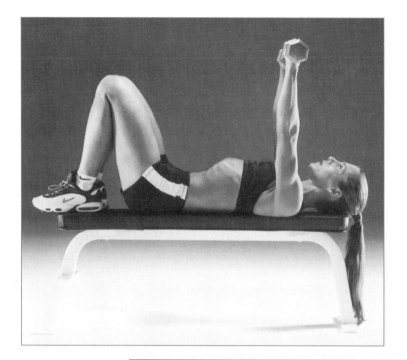

STARTING
POSITION

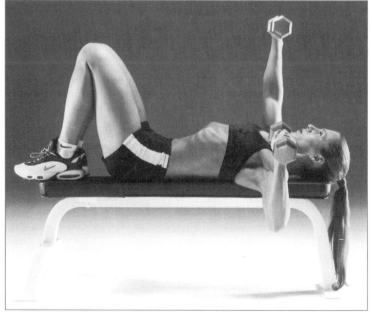

MOVEMENT

ONE-ARM DUMBBELL PRESS

This is one of Montel's favorite chest exercises. It requires strength, balance, and excellent coordination.

STARTING POSITION:

- Sitting on the end of a flat bench, grab two dumbbells.
- Rest the dumbbells on the tops of your thighs.
- Lie back on the bench, bringing both dumbbells up directly over your chest.

MOVEMENT:

- Press both dumbbells up in the air over your chest toward the ceiling.
- Contract both sides of your chest, remembering to hold your shoulders down while sticking your chest up.
- Keeping your left arm extended, focus on contracting the left side of your chest extra hard as you lower your right arm for a stretch. Lower your right arm as in the Dumbbell Press, and then press it back up to meet your left arm.
- Contract the right side of your chest extra hard while you now lower your left arm.

With any chest exercise, take three seconds to lower the weight, pause for one second at the stretched-out position, then take one second to lift it. The pause is important. You don't want the movement's momentum to do the work that your muscles are supposed to be doing.

WINI'S TRAINING TIP:

Don't forget to rest between sets. Your muscles need to rest and recover some of their blood supply before you challenge them again. How long should you rest between sets? If you're doing 8 to 12 reps of any exercise, resting one minute between sets is sufficient. Always go by how you feel. You should feel ready to begin the next set with intensity equal or beyond that of the previous set.

A word about intensity: You need to give your muscles a challenge. By doing so, they will adapt by growing stronger and then change into the muscles you want to see.

What does a challenge feel like to you? That's how intensely you should be working.

ℒ ℒ ℒ

CHAPTER 11

UpperBodyChange
Back

Back muscles need to be strong in order to carry us through this world with power. They're hard to see in the mirror and are often ignored in our training programs, yet they're a very important part of training—essential for good posture—and should not be neglected.

Have you ever seen a guy with well-developed biceps shuffling around the gym? You can tell he obviously works out and trains hard. He's developed a beautifully defined set of chest, arm, and abdominal muscles. Those are what I call the "ego" muscles—the ones you can see in a mirror. But by ignoring his back muscles—the ones that are more difficult to see—he can't really stand up straight enough to show off all that hard work. So back muscles are very important. One life lesson we can take from the effort to develop our back muscles is to pay attention to the things that aren't so obvious.

The back is made up of many muscle groups. We work them together because they're used in concert during many life activities. Besides the obvious latissimus dorsi, there's also the trapezius, rhomboids, and erector spinae. A big mistake people make is that they tend to use the arms to do the work that the back should. So, always initiate the movement at the shoulder girdle, where the shoulder blades, or scapula, are located. Remember to focus your attention on the back, and let the biceps just go for the ride. Don't pull with your arms first. Begin the movement from your back.

ONE-ARM DUMBBELL ROWS

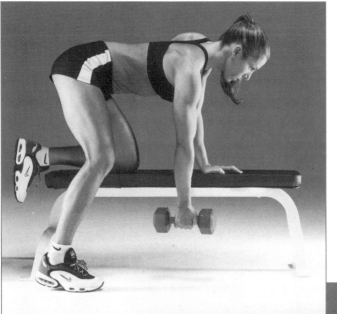

STARTING POSITION

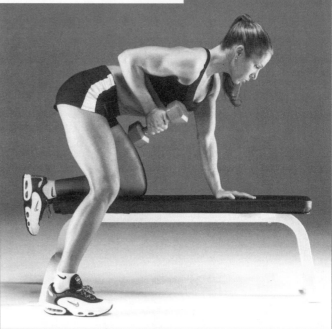

MOVEMENT

ONE-ARM DUMBBELL ROWS

STARTING POSITION:

- Kneel with your left knee on the bench and your right foot flat on the floor.
- Take a dumbbell in your right hand, and start with your arm extended toward the floor in a 6 o'clock position, but not locked at the elbow. Your palm is facing your body.

MOVEMENT:

- Initiate the movement by drawing your shoulder blades together toward the midline of your body as you move the weight, then draw your elbow up until the dumbbell reaches the height of your waist.
- Squeeze your upper back as you draw your elbow toward your hip.
- Remember to keep your elbows close to your body, as if you were squeezing a sponge in your upper back.
- Lower the dumbbell to the starting position.

REMEMBER:

- Square your hips and shoulders.
- Keep your back in a neutral position—don't move it. Move your arm from the shoulder blade.
- Draw in your abdominals.
- Look at the bench so your neck stays aligned.

BodyChange BONUS:

To vary the challenge, change the direction of your hand through the movement:

- Start with your palm facing rear.
- Rotate your arm as you bring the weight up so your palm faces your waist at the completion of the movement.

• ○ •

BENT-OVER DUMBBELL ROW

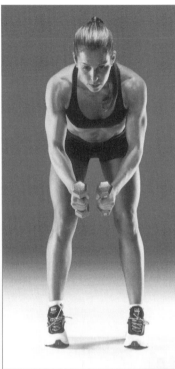

STARTING POSITION

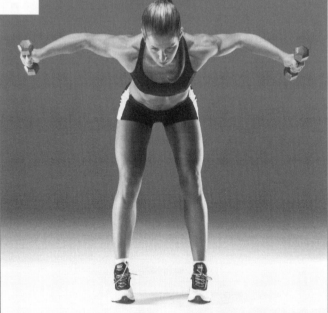

MOVEMENT

BENT-OVER DUMBBELL ROW

STARTING POSITION:

- Stand with your legs hip-width apart.
- Hold a lightweight dumbbell in each hand.
- Bend at your hips until your head is at 10 o'clock (where 9 o'clock would be parallel to the floor).
- Extend your arms toward the floor.

MOVEMENT:

- Draw your elbows out to your sides, creating a box, and keep your back flat and elongated.
- Draw your shoulder blades together, and contract your back muscles hard for a moment.
- Lower the weight slowly.

REMEMBER:

- Keep your back flat, not hunched.
- Use weights that are light enough so that you maintain control through the full range of the motion.
- Look slightly ahead at the floor to keep your neck aligned.

The bent-over dumbbell row works your upper back muscles, while the abdominals and lower back act as stabilizers.

❧ ❧ ❧

CHAPTER 12

UpperBodyChange
Shoulders

Chiseled, well-defined deltoids provide a great frame to your body. Well-developed shoulder muscles make the back appear wider and the waist appear smaller. Aesthetics aside, BodyChange demands that we strengthen every link in our body's muscle chain.

Our shoulders assist us with everything we do with our more powerful chest and back. They need to be strong to support the complicated challenges of life. We must take care of all the parts of our body, especially those that aren't as tough as others. We're only as strong as our weakest link.

Make sure you're warmed up for these exercises. By warming up first, we increase blood flow to the area and prepare it for the range of motion necessary to perform the exercises properly.

• • •

STANDING LATERAL RAISE

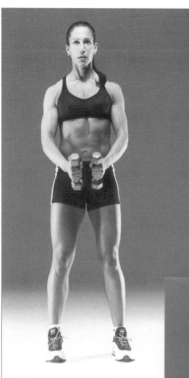

STARTING POSITION

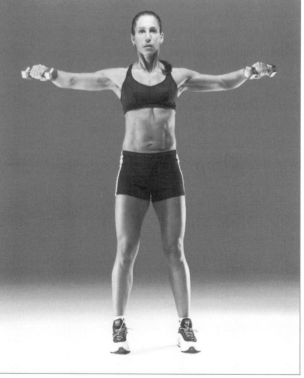

MOVEMENT

STANDING LATERAL RAISE

STARTING POSITION:

- Stand with your legs hip-width apart.
- Hold a light dumbbell in each hand, arms at your side, with your palms facing each other.
- Keep your arms slightly bent.

MOVEMENT:

- Raise your arms until they're parallel with the floor. Think about your arms traveling through a circular motion from 6 o'clock to 9 o'clock to 3 o'clock.
- Rotate your thumbs slightly down as you move, as if you're pouring a drop of water.
- Lower the weights in a slow, controlled motion.

REMEMBER:

- Hold your shoulders down as you lift your arms.
- Keep the rest of your body still. If you find that you're swinging your arms, you're using momentum, not muscles.

BODYCHANGE CHALLENGE:

If you perform this exercise while sitting on a Swiss ball, it will increase the balance challenge.

• • •

SEATED REAR LATERAL RAISE

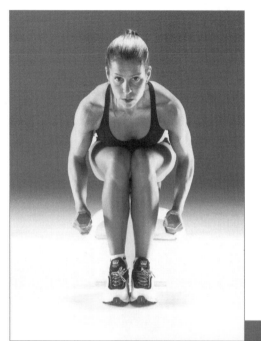

**STARTING
POSITION**

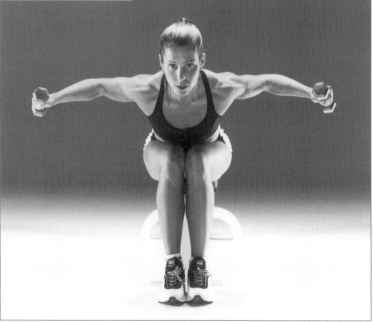

MOVEMENT

SEATED REAR LATERAL RAISE

STARTING POSITION:

- Sit on the end of a bench, with light dumbbells in each hand.
- Lean over, keeping your back elongated and your abdominals drawn.
- Your arms should be at the sides of your lower legs.

MOVEMENT:

- Lift your arms out to the side, squeezing your rear deltoids
  (the back of the shoulders) on top.
- Lower your arms with control.

This exercise is a variation of the rear lateral raise and is easier on your back. It removes the challenge from your legs and allows you to focus on your rear deltoids.

• • •

REAR LATERAL RAISE

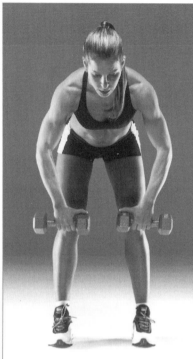

STARTING POSITION

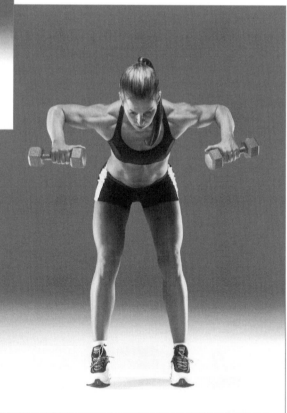

MOVEMENT

REAR LATERAL RAISE

This is my personal favorite—and Montel performs this exercise beautifully. The rear lateral raise works the often-neglected section of the back of your shoulders—the area that helps you hold your shoulders back so you can stand tall.

One of the keys to successful shoulder training is concentration. If you use too much weight or lapse into incorrect form, the larger muscle groups of the chest and back will do the work instead of the shoulder muscles. Therefore, you must feel your deltoids working when you do a lateral raise. Don't rush through it. Slow down and take the time to feel and understand what's going on with your body.

STARTING POSITION:

- Stand with your legs hip-width apart.
- Hold a light dumbbell in each hand.
- Bend at your hips, with no break at the waist.
  Your head is at 10 o'clock, where 9 o'clock would be parallel
  with the floor.
- Extend your arms toward the floor, keeping your
  elbows soft and your hands together.

MOVEMENT:

- Extend your arms out to the side until your hands are in line with
  your shoulders, then squeeze the back of your shoulders together.
- Slowly, with a controlled movement, lower your arms into their
  starting position.

REMEMBER:

- Always set up a shoulder exercise by pressing your shoulders down and drawing in your abdominals.
- Pause at the top of the movement (in a contracted position), as if trying to squeeze the last bit of water out of a sponge in your shoulder muscles.
- Take your time and savor this movement. Think about your arm traveling out to the side.
- Use the muscle, not momentum, to move the weight.

One of my clients, Janet, is a runner with strong legs and a powerful upper body, but it was clear when we first started working together that we needed to include a rear deltoid movement in every one of her shoulder workouts. She tended to slump over at the end of her long runs. I got her to do a basic deltoid lateral raise she'd read about in some of the fitness magazines.

Her shoulders are already strong on the sides and in the front from the chest exercises she did that helped develop her shoulders. Yet as a runner, we needed to build up the rear deltoids to balance out her posture. After we added the rear lateral raises, she can now run her races better, and she appears much taller than her 5'2" frame suggests.

Another client, Julia, stopped looking for suits with shoulder pads after we focused on her rear deltoids. She has a good frame, and although she's very small, she has great definition and is very fit. Her waist is trim, and her shoulders have great cuts in them. Throwing away her old clothes was never one of her training goals. Instead, we train together to feel strong and to give her a sense of control over how she feels. The buff appearance of this 54-year-old is a wonderful benefit of training for function.

ʓ ʓ ʓ

CHAPTER 13

UpperBodyChange
Triceps

We are forever flexing our very visible biceps, yet it's the triceps that take up two-thirds of the upper arm! The triceps are important because they assist us when we have to push something.

When one client of mine, Barbara, first started working with me several years ago, she said she didn't care about developing her triceps. She just wanted to eliminate the jiggle on the back of her upper arm. I took a very positive approach, teaching her about this muscle group and showing her how the jiggle could eventually be replaced with strong, lean muscle. She doesn't call her arms jiggly anymore. That jiggle disappeared as she decreased her body fat and developed her triceps.

Some of us may find the triceps difficult to feel during training because we can't see them easily when we're working them. Put one hand on the back of your upper arm and extend your elbow. Squeeze the back of your arm tightly. Those muscles are your triceps.

Montel has some of the most completely developed triceps I've ever seen. Many bodybuilders work their triceps for years without achieving the kind of definition he has in his upper arms. We constantly work his triceps from all angles, because this muscle has three heads and needs to be challenged in a number of different ways.

ONE-ARM TRICEPS KICKBACKS

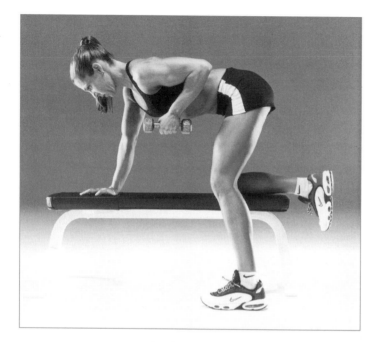

STARTING POSITION

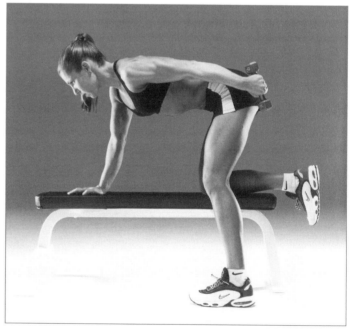

MOVEMENT

ONE-ARM TRICEPS KICKBACKS

Triceps kickbacks are a real treat for these muscles. It's relatively easy to feel this movement in the contracted position because, with your arm extended, you're working against gravity. This exercise isolates your triceps and is a great way to become familiar with the way they feel when they're contracted.

STARTING POSITION:

- Lean on a flat bench, placing one hand and knee on the bench for support.
- Keep your back neutral, your abdominals drawn, and your neck elongated.
- Hold a dumbbell in your free hand, and lift your elbow until it's slightly above the level of your back.
- Keep your upper arm close to the side of your body.

MOVEMENT:

- Keeping your upper arm still, extend your elbow from a position perpendicular to the floor, to parallel with the floor. In other words, your hand goes from the 6 o'clock position to the 3 o'clock position.
- Take an extra moment to fully contract your triceps when your arm is extended.
- Slowly return your hand back to the 6 o'clock position while keeping your upper arm still.
- Keep your palm facing your body.

REMEMBER:

- Keep your upper arm glued to your side. Imagine holding a $100 bill between your upper arm and the side of your body.
- Only move your elbow joint. Everything else remains still.
- Keep your back flat and neutral, with your shoulders and hips squared even, not moving.
- When you pause at the top of each repetition, imagine that you're squeezing water out of a sponge that's in the back of your arms.

BodyChange BONUS:

As your arm straightens, rotate your lower arm so that your palm is facing down at the end of the movement. This variation brings the focus to a different section of the triceps.

• • •

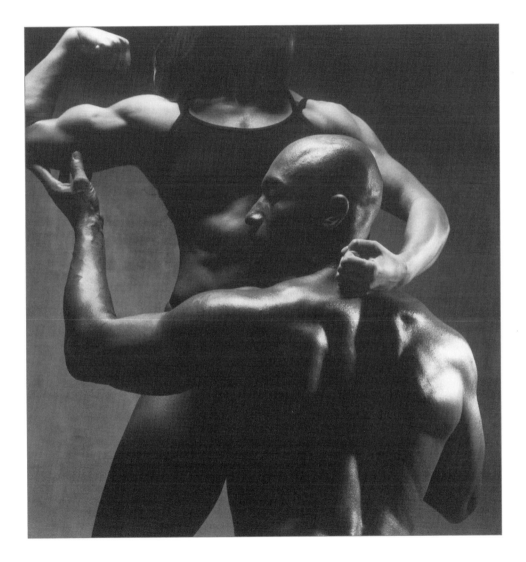

ONE-ARM SEATED TRICEPS EXTENSIONS

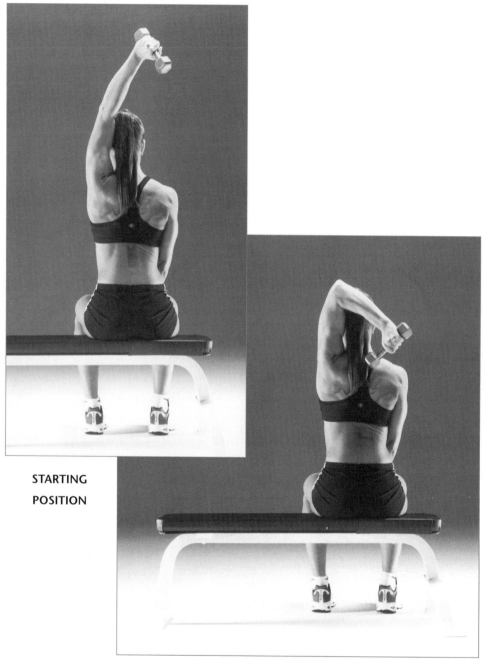

STARTING
POSITION

MOVEMENT

ONE-ARM SEATED TRICEPS EXTENSIONS

STARTING POSITION:

- Sit on the end of a bench, and press one light dumbbell overhead by extending your arm toward the ceiling.
- Place your palm so that it's facing forward.
- Position your upper arm so that it's right next to your ear.

MOVEMENT:

- Lower the dumbbell behind your head toward your opposite ear to the 5 o'clock position.
- Pause at the bottom, feeling the slight stretch in the triceps.
- Slowly extend your arm to the upward position.
- Visualize going from 12 o'clock when your arm is extended overhead, to 5 o'clock when your elbow is bent.
- Keep your neck elongated.

REMEMBER:

- Keep your back neutral, your shoulders down, and your neck elongated.
- Keep your elbow pointing upward.
- Be sure your upper arm remains right next to the side of your head.
- Keep your upper arm still, and move only your elbow joint.
- Do not hyperextend your elbow when you lengthen your arm.
- Always lower your arm slowly, keeping full awareness of where the weight is in relation to your head. Feel the stretch fully.
- Be sure to use a light dumbbell when doing this exercise the first few times.

BodyChange BONUS:

Try this exercise in a standing position to challenge your body awareness to an even greater extent.

• • •

This is one of my client Laura's favorite exercises. She loves the idea of a clock face, drawing the weight from 5 o'clock to 12 o'clock. If she is ever unsure of her range of motion, she remembers that the dumbbell needs to travel to 5 o'clock.

My client Jonathan, on the other hand, enjoys this exercise because he likes the way he can see the muscles in his triceps working while he bends his arm. The more controlled he keeps the movement while he's performing it, the better his arm appears. I always tell him to let the mirror be his guide: The better the form, the better his arm will look doing the exercise.

So look in the mirror—it tells you the truth.

☀ ☀ ☀

CHAPTER 14

UpperBodyChange
Biceps

"Make a muscle" is the first thing Montel's young son requested of me when I met him. Of course I instinctively flexed my biceps. Aside from impressing young children, biceps that are well developed make pulling weights and carrying our packages—excess baggage included—a whole lot easier.

• • •

STANDING DUMBBELL CURL

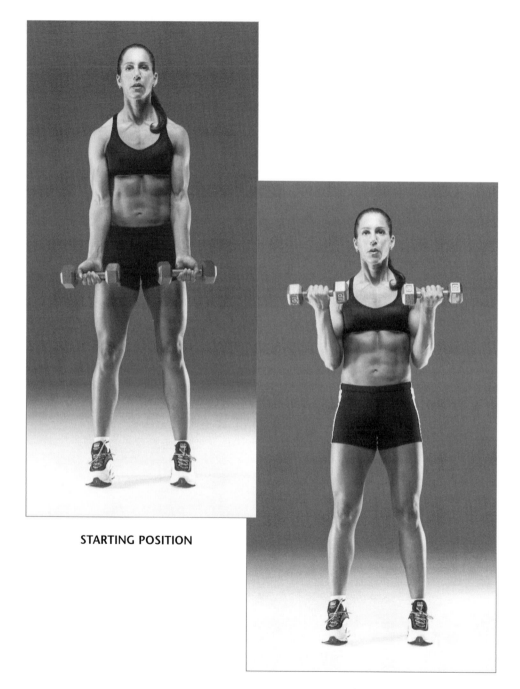

STARTING POSITION

MOVEMENT

STANDING DUMBBELL CURL

This is the meat-and-potatoes exercise of your biceps routine. Basic and efficient, it challenges your biceps to adapt to the workload it places on them. The beauty of using dumbbells is that even if both arms are moving at the same time, they're working independently.

STARTING POSITION:

- Stand with your legs hip-width apart.
- Hold a dumbbell in each hand.
- Extend your arms so that the dumbbells are down at your sides.
- Turn your palms so they face front.

MOVEMENT:

- Contract your biceps so that as you bend your elbows, you bring the dumbbells up toward your shoulders.
- Move your hands from the 6 o'clock position, or perpendicular to the floor, to the 11 o'clock position, or close to (but not touching) your shoulder.
- Lower your hands slowly, with control.

REMEMBER:

- Keep your upper arms close to the sides of the body as you move your lower arms. Imagine that you're holding a $100 bill between your arm and the side of your body.
- Hold your shoulders down as you lift your arms.
- Keep the rest of your body still. If you find yourself swinging, you're using momentum and not the muscle to throw the weight around. Keep the movement controlled.

BODYCHANGE BONUS:

Do this exercise one arm at a time. You can focus more fully on each arm.

BODYCHANGE CHALLENGE:

Do a drop set. Complete eight repetitions with a slightly heavier weight, then immediately pick up a lighter set of dumbbells and do another eight repetitions.

• • •

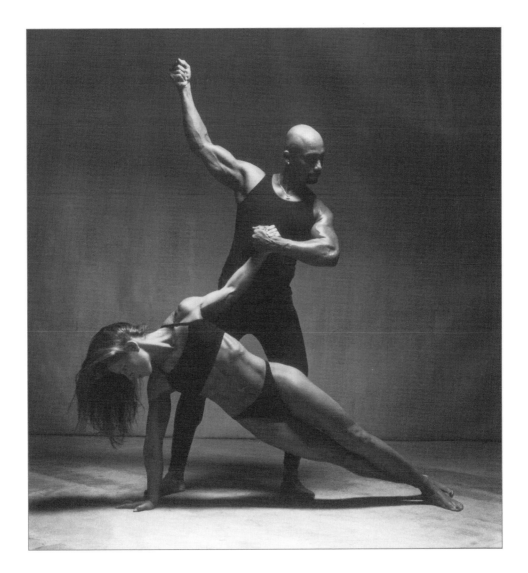

SEATED INCLINE DUMBBELL CURLS

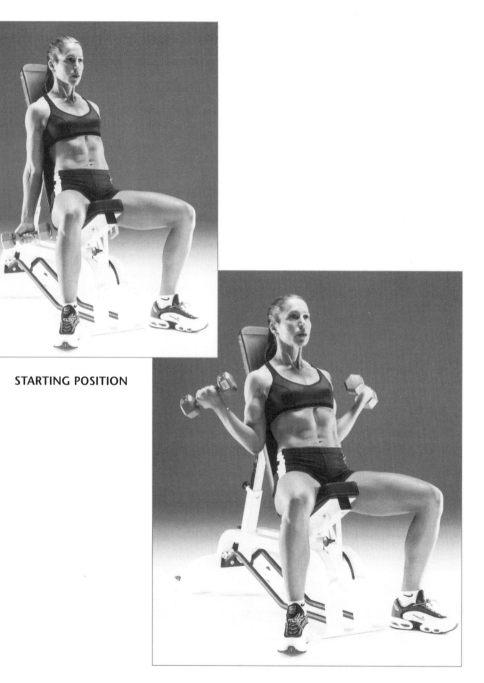

STARTING POSITION

MOVEMENT

SEATED INCLINE DUMBBELL CURLS

This exercise falls into the love-hate category. It's extremely challenging because it isolates the inner head of the biceps and focuses the fatigue in that one specific area. Ouch! Yet because it's so precise, it's easy to see your biceps working. Be sure to do this movement in front of a mirror. Let the visual feedback motivate you to go beyond your comfort zone.

STARTING POSITION:

- Sit on an incline bench set at a steep angle so that your body is at a 75- to 80-degree angle to the floor.
- Sit tall, with your back neutral and your feet securely on the floor.
- Hold a dumbbell in each hand, with your arms hanging down at your sides.
- Turn your palms so that they face forward.
- Keep your shoulders down and your neck elongated.

MOVEMENT:

- Keep your elbows close to your body as you draw the weight toward your shoulders.
- Let your pinkies lead the way, focusing on the inside head of the biceps.
- Take a moment at the top of the movement when the biceps are fully contracted.
- Lower the weight slowly.

REMEMBER:

- Make sure you do a full range of motion, yet be careful not to hyper-extend your elbows at the bottom of the movement.
- Visualize your biceps filling with air as you contract them.
- Keep the rest of your body still. The only movement is at the elbow joints.
- Lead with your little finger to target the inner head of your biceps.
- Be careful not to lean forward as you lift. Keep your back neutral.

BODYCHANGE BONUS:

Supersets are an advanced method of training. Try super-setting Standing Dumbbell Curls with Seated Incline Dumbbell Curls. Using a lighter weight and a slightly lower rep scheme of 8 to 10 reps, perform the two exercises rapidly in succession, allowing no more than three seconds between the two. This superset technique shocks the biceps and provides you with more of a BodyChange challenge. Imagine each repetition filling your biceps with power.

ℒ ℒ ℒ

CHAPTER 15

BodyChange
Abdominals

Strong abs are needed to support your lower back, make you less prone to injury, keep your posture erect by supporting your spine, and help you maintain good balance. Abdominals are so essential that they even help us laugh.

Strong abdominals imply a strong core. We need to have a solid center to rely on. Spiritually as well as physically, we must increase our capabilities by starting with our center.

Our midsection work consists of more than just one muscle group:

- **Rectus abdominus** runs from the pubic bone to the chest. Even though there's an abundance of information about abdominal training, and lots of references to either the upper of lower abs, they're actually part of the same muscle group, the rectus abdominus. It's what most people think of when they talk about abs, and it really is just one long muscle running from below the chest down into the pelvis.

- **External and internal obliques** are considered the muscles of the waistline. They both help you move diagonally.

- The **transverse abdominus** runs across the midsection.
  This muscle pulls the abdominal wall inward.

The abdominals are often misunderstood: We either concentrate on them as an afterthought to a workout, or they're worked on for too long without any real effort. The key to working your abs to get results is to be truly aware of each contraction. You need to feel each rep **in color.**

It's hard to believe, but you'll improve your abs gradually, and when you do, you'll feel stronger and more powerful than you do right now. Eventually you'll have to increase the challenge by choosing different and more difficult exercises. You can do this by increasing the angle of a decline bench, for example, or by adding resistance—such as increasing the weight or lever (angle). Montel sometimes lifts an eight-pound medicine ball with his feet when he does his reverse sit-ups on a bench. That's a real challenge to his already well-developed abs.

Remember: A chain is only as strong as its weakest link, and abdominals are the center of your strength. Don't let weak abdominals hold you back or prevent you from doing what you want or need to do. Build your wall of armor!

• • •

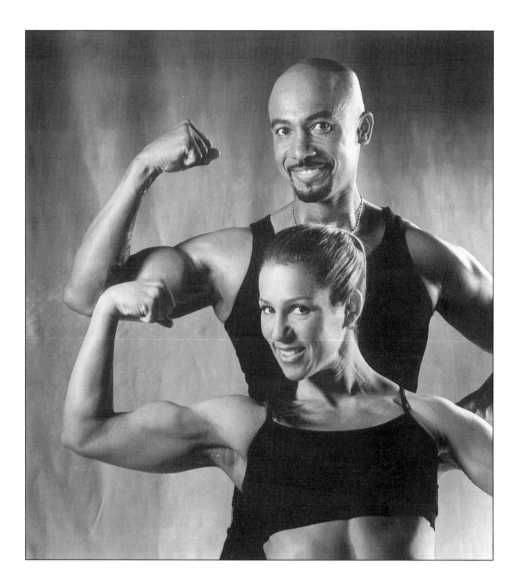

SWISS BALL CRUNCHES

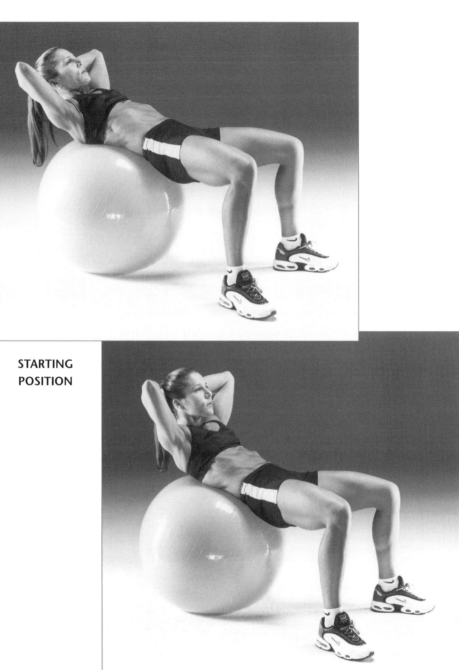

STARTING
POSITION

MOVEMENT

SWISS BALL CRUNCHES

Using a Swiss ball is a great way to challenge the entire range of motion of your abdominals. Your abdominals begin their range of motion 30 degrees to the rear, meaning that if you're lying flat on the floor, you're missing some of the stretch and contraction that abs are designed to do. Therefore, lying on a Swiss ball gives you a better range of motion than lying on the floor.

STARTING POSITION:

- Lie back on a Swiss ball, and drop your hips so that your lower back is totally supported.
- Place your hands on the sides of your head. Place your feet flat on the floor slightly more than hip-width apart for balance.
- Draw your abdominals in by scooping a bowl between your ribs and hips.

MOVEMENT:

- Contract your abdominals by pushing your ribs toward your hips.
- When your abdominals are fully contracted, draw them down as though scooping out a bowl in your center.
- Return to the starting position while keeping your abs tight.

REMEMBER:

- Concentrate on moving the middle of your spine, not your head and neck. Don't pull at your head or neck for extra "oomph"! Control this movement from your midsection, with your head merely going along for the ride.
- Keep your eyes glued to a point on the wall so your head doesn't yank around and throw you off balance on the Swiss ball.

BODYCHANGE **BONUS:**

Once you can balance this movement well on the Swiss ball, increase the challenge by placing your feet closer together on the floor, hugging a towel or a lightweight medicine ball between your knees.

BODYCHANGE **CHALLENGE:**

To increase the challenge of Swiss ball crunches, extend one arm directly behind you while keeping one hand behind or at the side of your head as you contract your abs. This position increases the lever, and therefore poses more challenge to your abdominal muscles.

• • •

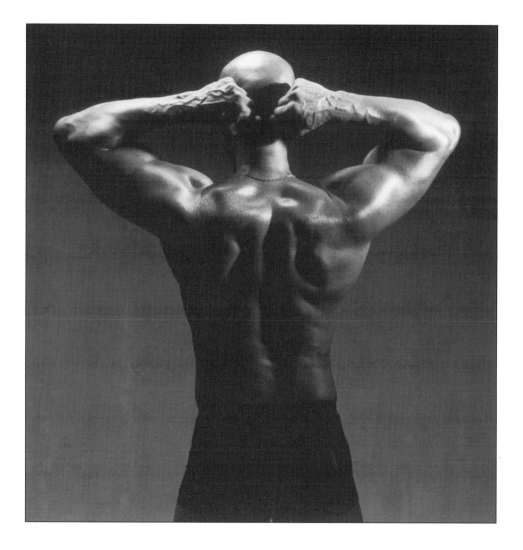

REVERSE CURLS

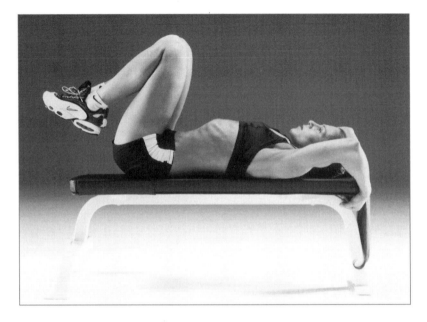

STARTING POSITION

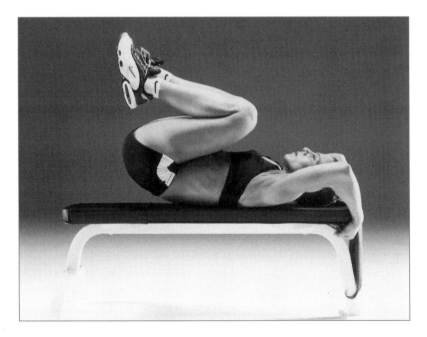

MOVEMENT

REVERSE CURLS

STARTING POSITION:

- Lie on your back on a flat bench.
- Hold on to the bench, with your arms as shown.
- Bend your knees, and then bend your legs upward so your knees are in line with your hips.

Option: *Place a towel between your bent knees to help you connect to the lower section of your abdominals.*

MOVEMENT:

- Draw your abdominals in and back as you roll your pelvis toward your ribs. (Think about decreasing the distance between your ribs and hips.)
- Visualize making a bowl with your abdominals as you curl your hips toward your rib cage.
- Draw your knees from a 12 o'clock starting position to a 10 o'clock ending position.
- Pause at the top of the movement to hold your contracted position before lowering.

REMEMBER:

- Keep constant tension in your abdominals by taking an extra moment to feel them in the contracted position.

BODYCHANGE BONUS:

Reverse curls are challenging, but once your abs have adapted, use a light medicine ball instead of a towel to add resistance to the exercise.

• • •

HIP RAISE (ADVANCED)

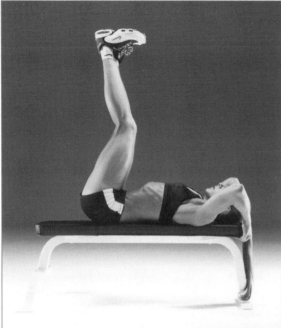

STARTING POSITION

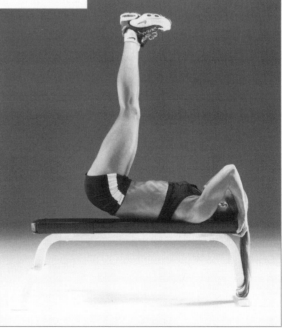

MOVEMENT

HIP RAISE (ADVANCED)

STARTING POSITION:

- Lie flat on your back on a bench.
- Hold on to the bench as shown.
- Extend your legs up into the air, with your knees slightly bent.

Option: *Place a towel in between your knees to help you connect to your abdominals.*

MOVEMENT:

- Draw your abs in and back. This movement will raise your hips up off the bench and toward your ribs. Remember to keep your legs extended into the air.
- Hold your hips up for one moment, then gently lower them to the bench.

REMEMBER:

- Scoop your abdominals like a bowl as you do *each* repetition.
- Stay super-aware of your abdominals, drawing *down* as your hips raise just an inch or two off the bench. This exercise is a tiny movement that packs a punch.
- Visualize your hips moving from the 9 o'clock to the 10 o'clock position.

• • •

DIAGONAL CRUNCH

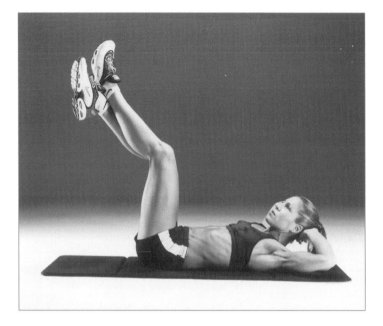

STARTING POSITION

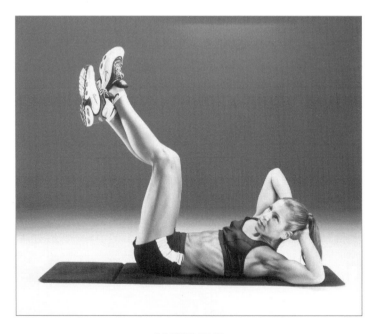

MOVEMENT

DIAGONAL CRUNCH

This exercise strengthens the abdominals and the obliques, the muscles of the waistline.

STARTING POSITION:

- Lie on the floor on your back, with legs up, knees bent, and ankles crossed.
- Place your hands behind your head.

MOVEMENT:

- Leading with your left side, draw your left rib and shoulder toward your right knee. Remember to keep your elbow back.
- Slowly lower your left side back to the floor, keeping constant tension in your abdominal muscles.
- Repeat this exercise toward the same side 15 times.
- Switch sides.

BODYCHANGE BONUS:

Increase the challenge by increasing the lever: Extend one arm over your head, then repeat the diagonal crunch movement. Be sure that your other arm supports your head.

ℒ ℒ ℒ

CHAPTER 16

Stretching

Montel: *Stretching helps me feel my body in a different way. I know that the more I stretch, the better I'll be able to work all those muscles I've built in the gym.*

• • •

The best time to stretch is after a workout, when the muscles are warm. Stretching should be a part of every workout. After you've completed your aerobics and weight-training workouts, take time to stretch out the muscles you've been training. The stretches relax the muscles that have tightened during your workout by drawing blood to them. Increased blood flow to the area helps to remove the toxins that have built up there during your workout.

Stretching helps you view your body in a different manner. When you stretch, you truly need to quiet your mind and imagine your muscles lengthening. We rush and run and power our way through each day, so can't we take a moment to slow down?

How should the stretches feel?

Comfortably uncomfortable. Remember: Stretch, not strain.

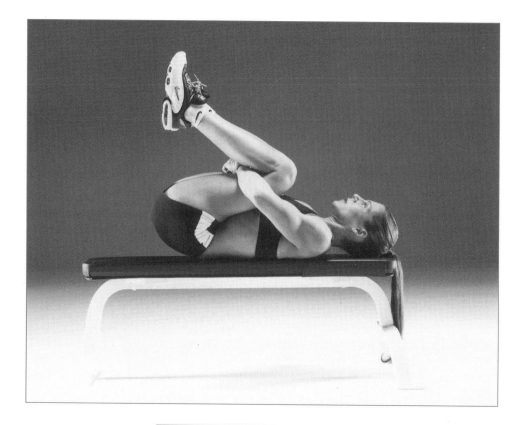

LOWER BACK STRETCH

This stretch opens up and relaxes the lower back.

STARTING POSITION:

• Lie on your back on a bench or a mat on the floor.

MOVEMENT:

• Gently hug your knees into your chest. In this position, think about your lower back opening up. Hold for a count of 10.

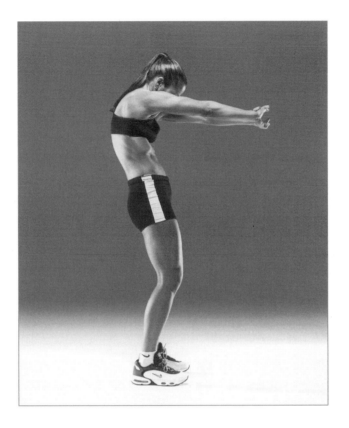

UPPER BODY STRETCH

This stretch relaxes the neck and upper back after working out or sitting too long at your computer.

STARTING POSITION:

- Standing in a neutral position, lace your fingers together, then turn them out with your palms facing away from you.

MOVEMENT:

- Reach forward, opening up your shoulder blades as you do. Keep your head down. Hold the stretch for a count of 10.

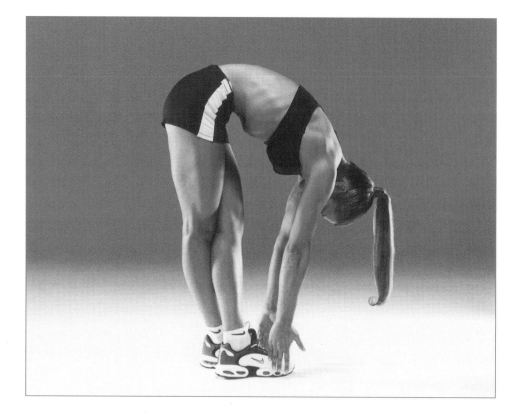

HAMSTRING STRETCH

STARTING POSITION:

- Standing in a neutral position, cross one leg behind the other.

MOVEMENT:

- Bend at your hips so that your arms hang down toward your feet.
- Hold for a count of 10.
- Place one hand on the front of your knee as you come up.
- Switch to stretch the other side.

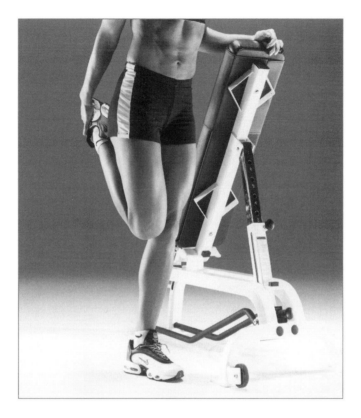

QUADRICEPS STRETCH

This movement is good for stretching out the front thigh muscles that get tight doing squats, aerobics, cycling, and lunges.

STARTING POSITION:

- Hold on to an incline bench or the back of a chair.

MOVEMENT:

- Standing on one foot, bend your opposite knee behind you, and with your hand, draw your heel into your rear so that you feel the stretch in your frontal thigh.
- Make sure your hips, knees, and shoulders are squared.
- Keep the leg you're standing on slightly bent.
- Hold for a count of 10.
- Lower your leg and switch.

℘ ℘ ℘

CHAPTER 17

Designing
Your Program

ow that you've read through the exercises, you're ready to develop a program that's right for your fitness level. Following are three basic programs: beginner, intermediate, and advanced. Use them as the basic foundation for your program. Modify them with the BodyChange bonuses described in the exercise section as you progress. The main focus here is to consistently follow one of the three basic programs. I've set it up so that you weight-train Monday, Wednesday, and Friday; add aerobics on Tuesday, Thursday, and Saturday; and then rest on Sunday. You can modify this to your schedule and choose another day off if you like.

If you've never worked out or are more than 30 pounds overweight, ease into the beginner program. Do one set of each exercise and see how you feel the next day. It might take a week or so to be able to complete the full routine six days in a row. You'll know the difference between being sore and being *really sore*. If you do get really sore (I'm talking about having trouble sitting down or standing up from a chair), then skip a day or two of weight training and just do your aerobics. Just keep moving. Don't worry. Beginners will see benefits faster than the experienced athlete. The body has an uncanny way of snapping to attention when it's put into motion.

• • •

BEGINNER PROGRAM

Warm-up: 15 minutes of movement

1. **Dumbbell Squat with Swiss Ball**   3 sets of 10 repetitions
2. **Walking Lunge**   3 sets of 10 steps
3. **Standing Calf Raise**   3 sets of 10 repetitions
4. **Beginner Push-Ups**   3 sets of 10 repetitions
5. **One-Arm Rows**   3 sets of 10 repetitions each arm
6. **Lateral Raise**   3 sets of 10 repetitions
7. **One-Arm Triceps Kickback**   3 sets of 10 repetitions each arm
8. **Dumbbell Curl**   3 sets of 10 repetitions each arm
9. **Swiss Ball Crunches**   3 sets of 20 repetitions

Stretching: Do each stretch—Lower Back, Upper Body, Hamstring, and Quadriceps—twice, holding each for 10 seconds.

Aerobics: Do 20 to 30 minutes at 65 to 75 percent maximum heart rate three times per week, ideally with a day of rest in between.

INTERMEDIATE PROGRAM

Warm-up: 15 minutes of movement

1.	**Dumbbell Squat**	3 sets of 12 repetitions
2.	**Step-Ups**	3 sets of 12 repetitions each leg
3.	**Walking Lunge**	3 sets of 12 steps
4.	**Standing Calf Raise**	3 sets of 12 repetitions each leg
5.	**Incline Dumbbell Press**	3 sets of 12 repetitions
6.	**Push-Ups**	3 sets of 12 repetitions
7.	**One-Arm Row**	3 sets of 12 repetitions each arm
8.	**Rear Lateral Raise**	3 sets of 12 repetitions
9.	**One-Arm Triceps Extension**	3 sets of 12 repetitions each arm
10.	**Seated Incline Dumbbell Curl**	3 sets of 12 repetitions
11.	**Swiss Ball Crunches**	3 sets of 25 repetitions
12.	**Reverse Sit-Ups**	3 sets of 15 repetitions

Stretching: Do each stretch—Lower Back, Upper Body, Hamstring, and Quadriceps—twice, holding each stretch for 10 seconds.

Aerobics: Do 30 to 40 minutes at 65 to 80 percent maximum heart rate three times per week, ideally with a day of rest in between.

℈ ℈ ℈

ADVANCED PROGRAM

Warm-up: 15 minutes of movement

1.	**Dumbbell Squat**	3 sets of 12 repetitions
2.	**Step-Ups**	3 sets of 12 repetitions each leg
3.	**Walking Lunge**	3 sets of 12 steps
4.	**Standing Calf Raise**	3 sets of 12 repetitions each leg
5.	**Incline Dumbbell Press**	3 sets of 10 repetitions
6.	**Push-Up on Swiss Ball**	3 sets of 10 repetitions
7.	**Bent-Over Dumbbell Rows**	3 sets of 10 repetitions
8.	**One-Arm Row**	3 sets of 10 repetitions each arm
9.	**Rear Lateral Raise**	3 sets of 10 repetitions
10.	**One-Arm Triceps Kickback**	3 sets of 10 repetitions each arm
11.	**One-Arm Triceps Extension**	3 sets of 10 repetitions each arm
12.	**Seated Incline Dumbbell Curl**	3 sets of 12 repetitions
13.	**Swiss Ball Crunches**	3 sets of 25 repetitions
14.	**Hip Raises**	3 sets of 15 repetitions

Stretching: Do each stretch—Lower Back, Upper Body, Hamstring, and Quadriceps—twice, holding each stretch for 10 seconds.

Aerobics: Do 30 to 45 minutes at 65 to 80 percent maximum heart rate three times per week, ideally with a day of rest in between.

℔ ℔ ℔

CHAPTER 18

Eating Smarter for Life

Montel: *I like my treats like everyone else, but the main thing I've learned over the years is to make sure I eat enough protein and smart carbohydrates to fuel me throughout my day. Wini usually asks me what I ate the previous day because she knows how I often go nonstop. I take the time—even when I'm very busy—to make sure I eat a protein-filled meal every couple of hours.*

• • •

The diet industry is huge, and diets are something that most of us are either going on or off. We need healthy eating habits to support us in our lives. It comes down to being aware, being consistent—and being smart.

What Are Your Goals?

I often hear from people who understand the basics of what healthy eating is about, yet still can't seem to lose those last five pounds or layer of body fat. It's so easy to become confused by the conflicting information. I see so many gym members gobbling up a high-sugar energy bar before their workouts, but that's often no better than a regular candy bar. It's a common sight—the gym members who grab bagels because they're fat free and blueberry muffins because they're sugar free—and hey, they're being sold at a health-food store so they *must* be good for you.

Well, I certainly don't think a bagel is *bad* for you. It's not going to lead to a heart attack or load your arteries up with cholesterol. Yet for many people, especially those who are trying to lose fat, it's the difference between being just all right and being lean and at your best. It always goes back to the question: *What are your goals?*

If you stay aware of your decisions regarding food, maintaining a healthful diet is not so difficult. We must exercise our awareness in the same way we exercise our muscles. The more we use it, the stronger our awareness gets.

Eating right for life should be a plan that works for you and your individual goals. Eating correctly is never about being hungry. Eating for life is never about being deprived. *True deprivation means not giving yourself the opportunity to take care of your body.*

We Can Control What We Eat

There are so many things in this world we can't control. But we *can* control what we put into our bodies. We can choose what to eat, and we can choose what not to eat. Of course there's a lot of conflicting information out there that can be very confusing, but it's up to you to take care of yourself. We need to define what we can control, what we can change, and the factors we need to work around.

We can't always change our work hours, so we adapt to that by scheduling a time to exercise that's convenient. Yet we can control the awareness and intelligent planning we bring to our workout sessions.

We may not be able to control the fact that we can't get home to cook lunch and dinner. Yet we can control the planning and preparation it takes to cook ahead and carry our meals with us.

When we become clear about the factors in our life we *can* control, and let go of the items we cannot, we will experience a great sense of relief.

Most people I speak with have the best of intentions. Unfortunately, they're overwhelmed by the huge amount of conflicting information they're bombarded with regarding weight loss. There is no *one* perfect diet. People have different metabolisms that respond in different ways. We are all different ages, at different levels of fitness, with different short- and long-term goals.

If you want a change, you have to *make* a change. If you do what you've always done, you will get what you've always gotten. Again: *What are your goals?*

Diet: Beyond Maintenance

Think of food as an energy source that needs to be on constant supply. Notice I said "energy source," not "high-carbohydrate source."

When I first started teaching classes, I was told to "eat carbs; carbs will give you energy." That was true then and it's true now, but the problem was that most instructors were eating too *many* carbs and too little protein. Eating carbohydrates cause the body to secrete the hormone insulin. Insulin converts carbohydrates to glycogen and stores it in the muscles and liver. From there, it's available to burn as energy. Glycogen is the first energy supply the body can use. Yet our bodies can only store so much of this type of energy. The rest gets stored as fat.

Also, eating too many carbohydrates at once causes your blood sugar to swing up, then crash down. That's why you're often tired after eating too many sweets. If you've read the latest research, the high-carbohydrate, eat-pasta-till-you-drop approach isn't the most effective one for many people. Elite athletes have been shown to perform better on a higher protein/lower carb diet. There is always that consistent gym exerciser who can't budge their body-fat level. This diet, or, better word—*attitude*—works best for them.

Of course, some people *can* lose weight eating pasta. Some people smoke for 50 years and never get lung cancer, too. But as far as you're concerned, forget about the supermodel who eats pizza and chain smokes. Forget about the guy training next to you who's afraid to do aerobics because he might lose too much weight. Let's learn from our own past history and experience. Get to know how your body responds to dietary changes. Don't compare yourself to the supermodels—they're aliens, did you know that? *Focus on what's going to work for you.*

Eat healthy. Eat smart. Listen to your body. Be aware. There's a wealth of information out there. Yet the most intelligent of us can still reach for foods that aren't healthful. Glazed doughnuts aren't going to do anything for you—except maybe hurt your sense of self. Try to stay away from foods high in sugar and fat. Chicken, fish, and lean meats; vegetables and fresh fruits; low-fat dairy products—build your eating plan around *those* items. Notice how you feel so your energy doesn't go on a roller-coaster ride.

Easy Access

Easy access is the key to eating healthfully. Plan ahead so that the right choices are accessible to you. That may entail cooking for the week over the weekend. It may mean researching restaurants before you frequent them. You need to have healthful foods accessible to you so you won't be in a situation where you grab something that's not good for you because nothing else is available.

My client Alice prepares her whole week's worth of snacks on Sunday nights. She usually has a protein shake for breakfast and orders in some steamed vegetables for lunch, which she throws a can of tuna on. She keeps her refrigerator stocked with healthful choices that she prepares ahead of time. When she gets home from a long day, her meal of broiled chicken and salad is already precooked. She has no need to grab something quick and fried, for she knows she has a quick, nutritious meal waiting at home.

Tips for Smart Eating:

- Try to "get fresh" whenever possible. Fresh fruits and vegetables are full of fiber and nutrients.

- Avoid processed meats. They're full of sugar, salt, and ingredients you don't even want to know about.

- Drink plenty of water. Keep a bottle on your desk and in your car. Don't wait until you're thirsty. Keep the water coming in.

- Get into the habit of cooking a bunch of chicken breasts at once. Wrap them individually in aluminum foil so they can be a quick snack, cold or hot.

- Nonfat yogurt can be a great sweet treat. Mix it with some cold berries if you're having a cookie panic.

- Make sure you always have something to eat when you get home. Don't wait until you're tired and hungry to start shopping or cooking.

- Keep some easy-access snacks such as hard-boiled eggs or cut-up vegetables ready in the refrigerator.

When I get home at night, the first thing I do is throw some frozen vegetables in the microwave. While they're cooking, I either put some fresh fish on the broiler or start slicing some already prepared chicken breast. If for some reason I don't have chicken or fresh fish around, I always make sure I have some eggs boiled (I boil them two dozen at a time), or I open a can of tuna.

Breakfast

Breakfast is an important meal and should include protein just like every other meal. If you don't like to eat first thing in the morning, that's fine. However, when you do have your first meal of the day, remember that you're fueling your body with good, healthful food to propel you through the day.

Suggested breakfast choices:

- Low or nonfat yogurt
- Oatmeal with egg whites
- Protein shake with protein powder and fresh fruit
- Low-fat cottage cheese

Lunch

Lunch is often taken on the run. If you prepare your food at home, now is the time to break out that chicken breast and steamed broccoli. Or perhaps try a medley of vegetables with fish or turkey. Remember: Eat protein and smart carbohydrates.

Suggested lunch choices:

- Chicken and salad
- Steamed shrimp and broccoli
- Turkey on whole grain/high-fiber bread with lettuce and tomato

Dinner

Make sure it's easy-access. Have that nutritious food available to you when you get home. Try a variety of vegetables, various kinds of fish, or your chicken cooked a different way. Keep the protein and vegetables coming in.

Suggested dinner choices:

- Stir-fry (in a nonstick pan) chicken, peppers, and onions; and serve with a baked potato
- Grill fish with some balsamic vinegar; serve with steamed asparagus
- Sear a lean steak and serve with salad

Ways That Meals Don't "Count":

- If I eat it fast
- If I eat while driving
- If my grandmother made it

- If it's a holiday
- If it's my birthday
- If it's my sister's birthday
- If it's my sister's best friend's brother's birthday
- If it's fat free (fat-free foods are often loaded with sugar; this country has gotten fat on fat-free!)
- If it's eaten in the movies—so the candy and popcorn don't count
- If I have it at a coffee bar (I'll have a double mocha frozen coffee drink with whipped cream—but it's bought at a coffee bar, so it doesn't count)
- If I'm at a meeting and everyone is eating doughnuts
- If I bought some cookies at a health-food store and they're preservative free

Remember: *Everything counts.*

You're certainly allowed to make conscious decisions regarding special occasions and holidays. After all, *you* are in charge of your life—this is your ride. Yet if you *do* decide on that piece of cake, please eat it with awareness—don't gobble it down or eat it while you're driving. Enjoy it! Eating that one piece of cake won't do as much harm as eating everything else on the dessert tray because you feel so bad about yourself.

Stay aware, stay conscious—and enjoy your birthday (and every other day) by treating yourself with love and respect!

ℒ ℒ ℒ

AFTERWORD

"What we hope ever to do with ease,
we must learn first to do with diligence."
— Samuel Johnson (British author, 1709-1784)

This program sounds great, but how do I stick with it?

Here are some tips to help you do just that:

- Make the commitment to give this program your best shot. It takes 21 days to develop a habit—accept the challenge of those 21 days. Training is always challenging, yet your interpretation of it will change as it becomes a part of your daily life.

- Accept that it may be difficult to begin; however, it's more difficult to stay in the same place.

- Check in with a friend or family member. Human beings need support. Share your goals with someone you trust. Call that person when you lose sight of your goals.

- Plan your work—and work your plan. Make an appointment with yourself for your workout. Write it in your schedule. Treat that appointment with the respect with which you treat your other commitments. The better you take care of yourself, the better you'll be able to honor all your commitments.

- Log your workouts. Go over your past training records. Recall how good you felt when you finished a workout.

- Don't overanalyze why you're having a rough time beginning. Every journey starts with the first step—no matter how long that journey is.

- Remember: *This is your ride.* Your life. Your body. Your decisions. You're the one who can make a change. The hardest part will be those first two days. So for 21 days, accept that you'll be in unexplored territory.

- *You* are in control of the decisions you make. *You* are responsible for your choices. When you feel that the chocolate is choosing *you*, take control.

- You'll find that once you commit yourself to change, the whole world works with you. Of course, a lot of it has to do with the spin, or the interpretation, you put on things. When you realize that exercise is a gift you give yourself, it becomes a time you'll look forward to. It's a time that you'll take for *you—and* when you understand how good it makes you feel, adhering to it becomes easier.

- Exercise works. It changes lives, not just bodies. Learn that you have control over how you look and feel. It's not just your body that becomes stronger by following this program. The strength you acquire will support you in all aspects of your life.

Don't let your mind get in your way.

Remember: No one feels confident *all* the time.

We wish you all the best!

— Wini and Montel

ɞ ɞ ɞ

• About the Authors •

Montel Williams is the Emmy Award–winning host of the nationally syndicated *Montel* show. As a highly decorated former Naval intelligence officer, motivational speaker, actor, and humanitarian, Williams is an example of personal achievement for people throughout the country. He is the author of *Mountain, Get Out of My Way* and *Life Lessons and Reflections,* co-author of *Practical Parenting,* and the proud father of four children.

• • •

Wini Linguvic, the creator of BodyChange™, is one of New York's most sought-after personal trainers. She has more than 16 years experience designing fitness programs for the city's busiest people. Her clientele ranges from novices to fitness instructors. Wini has been featured on CBS News, as well as in *Vogue* and *Women's Sports and Fitness* magazines. She has been training Montel for the past five years. Website: **www.BodyChange.com**

ℓ ℓ ℓ

ፘ ፘ ፘ

We hope you enjoyed
this Mountain Movers Press/Hay House book.
If you would like to receive additional information, please contact:

c/o Hay House, Inc.
P.O. Box 5100
Carlsbad, CA 92018-5100

(760) 431-7695 or **(800) 654-5126**
(760) 431-6948 (fax) or **(800) 650-5115 (fax)**

Please visit the Hay House Website at: **hayhouse.com**

ፘ ፘ ፘ